Cafer's Antidepressants:
Visualize to Memorize™

First Edition, 2020

Author: Jason Cafer, MD

Editor: Julianna Link, PA-C

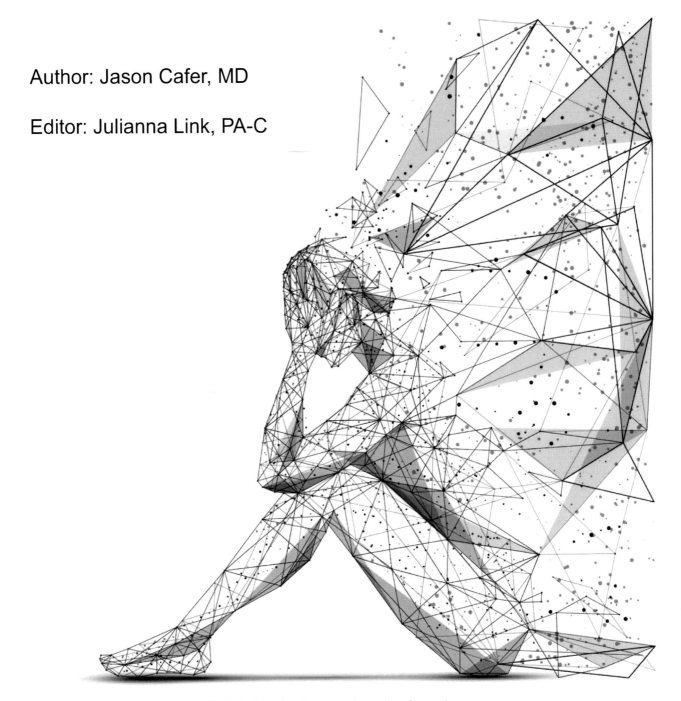

Cafer's Antidepressants: Visualize to Memorize

First Edition

Copyright 2020, CaferMed LLC

Author: Jason Cafer, MD

Editor: Julianna Link, PA-C

Illustrations: Coccus from 99Designs

Cover design: BengsWorks from 99Designs

Licensed images: Shutterstock and Wikimedia Commons

ISBN: 978-1-7350901-3-9

Contact: jasoncafer@gmail.com

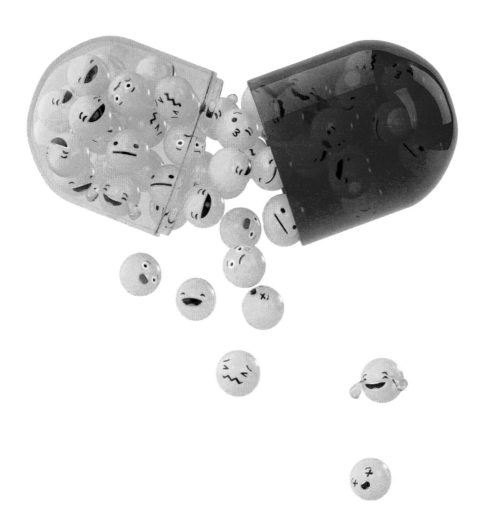

The scope of drug interaction information is limited to what can be digested and applied to routine clinical practice. There are countless unmentioned drug-drug interactions that could be relevant for some patients but are omitted because the amount of material would be overwhelming.

This book is focused on medications, not overarching psychiatric care. Although chemicals are necessary for treatment of mania or acute psychosis, pharmacologic treatment of depression/anxiety/insomnia/etc is not always the best medicine. Always consider interventions including cognitive behavioral therapy, diet, exercise, mindfulness, sleep hygiene, etc.

Dosing recommendations are for healthy adults, and may differ from FDA prescribing guidelines. Refer to other sources for treatment of children, older adults, pregnancy/breastfeeding and renal/hepatic insufficiency.

Every effort has been made to provide accurate and up-to-date information. Author/editors/publisher/reviewers disclaim all liability for direct or consequential damages resulting from the use of this material. Readers are encouraged to confirm information with other sources before incorporating it into your prescribing practice. Information should be compared with official instructions from the drug manufacturer.

Table of Contents

Fluvoxamine (Luvox) is a strong 1A2 inhibitor.

Citalopram, escitalopram, and sertraline are SSRIs metabolized by 2C19.

Fluoxetine, paroxetine, bupropion, and duloxetine are 2D6 inhibitors.

Most antidepressants are serotonergic.

Except for tricyclics, QT prolongation is rarely dangerous with antidepressants.

Some TCAs are anxiety-reducing, while others are drive-enhancing. All are 2D6 substrates.

Amitriptyline is strongly serotonergic and anticholinergic.

Several noradrenergic TCAs have so little serotonergic activity that they *could* be safely combined with an MAOI.

Sertraline is the preferred antidepressant during pregnancy.

Fluvoxamine is approved for OCD, not for depression.

Milnacipran (Savella) is an SNRI approved for fibromyalgia, not for depression.

Trazodone is commonly prescribed at low dose for insomnia, rarely prescribed at full antidepressant strength.

Mirtazapine (Remeron) is great for promoting sleep and stimulating appetite.

Atomoxetine (Strattera) is approved for ADHD, not for depression.

Esketamine nasal spray is for treatment-resistant depression.

Brexanolone is an intravenous neurosteroid approved for post-partum depression.

Some opioids can contribute to serotonin syndrome

Cyproheptadine is an antihistamine that blocks 5-HT2 serotonin receptors. It is used off-label for nightmares and to stimulate appetite.

Medication Monographs

#40 most prescribed (U.S.)
1993
$4–$250

Chemical structure

Generic Name (TRADE NAME)
pronunciation
mnemonic phrase

❖ Class of medication
❖ Mechanism of action

100
<u>200</u>
400
mg

Year the drug was introduced to the U.S. market

Monographs focus on the unique aspects of the individual drug, to be considered in context of the medication class. Most of the medications in this book are <u>psychotropic</u>, i.e., capable of affecting the mind, emotions and behavior.

Price range for a <u>month's supply</u> of the generic (if available) version of the drug. The price is generally applicable to the most commonly dispensed prescription, which would be #30 for drugs usually dosed QD, #60 for those dosed BID, and #90 for those usually dosed TID. The applicable milligram strength (200 mg in this example) is the number underlined in the upper righthand corner.

The bottom dollar value is the lowest GoodRx price, available with a coupon at select pharmacies. The high dollar value is the average retail price circa 2019–2020. The wide cost differential between pharmacies underscores the importance of checking <u>GoodRx</u> before filling a script for cash. For instance, #30 of olanzapine 20 mg was <u>$843 at Walgreens</u> ($276 with coupon) but only <u>$9 at Walmart</u> (Sept 2020).

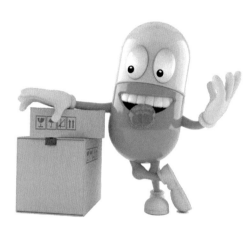

Each monograph features a mascot designed to pair the drug's generic name with the most common U.S. trade name.

A representative pill of the underlined strength, either a branded or generic version. The main purpose is to show whether we're talking capsules or tablets. For tablets, we try to show the side with score lines. If no score lines are shown, assume that the pill is not intended to be split. For any splittable psychotropic medication, giving a half dose for the first two days may be a good idea, depending on acuity of symptoms. <u>Cutting tablets in half can cut prescription cost in half</u> because a 20 mg tab is usually no more expensive than a 10 mg tab.

Dosing: When provided, dosing recommendations are applicable to healthy adults. Refer to other sources for pediatric recommendations. Older adults should generally be given lower doses. Doses may need to be modified when considering kinetic/dynamic interactions, pharmacogenetics, body weight, and renal/hepatic insufficiency. ePocrates.com and the free <u>ePocrates</u> app provide provide renal/hepatic dosing info.

Boxes like this contain contextual information about the drug.

A link to a page with relevant content looks like this:

3A4 substrate

The box with rounded corners contains a visual hybrid of the mascot and CYP interaction mnemonic(s). Over half of prescription drugs are metabolized by 3A4, so there are plenty of fish.

Recurring Visuals

  Antidepressant (rain cloud)

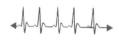 QT interval-prolonging medication

  Tricyclic antidepressant (TCA)

  Anticholinergic with CNS effects (Mad as a hatter)

  MAOI inhibitor (Chairman MAO)

  Antihistamine (push pin) - "anti-hiss-tamine"

4

PHARMACODYNAMICS VS PHARMACOKINETICS

Drug-drug interactions fall into two main categories: **pharmacokinetic** and **pharmacodynamic**.

Pharmacodynamics is what a drug does to the body. Pharmacodynamic interactions are based on the drugs' mechanisms of action and do not involve alteration in blood levels of either interacting drug.

Pharmacokinetics is what the body does to a drug. Kinetic derives from the Greek verb *kinein*, "to move". In this case we're talking movement into and out of the body, for instance absorbing the chemical from the gut and processing it for excretion in urine or feces. Pharmacokinetic (PK) interactions are generally manifested by alteration of blood levels of one of the interacting drugs.

For simplicity's sake, let's drop the *pharmaco-* prefix and refer to these concepts as **kinetic** interactions and **dynamic** interactions.

PHARMACODYNAMIC INTERACTIONS

Dynamic interactions are intuitive if you understand how the interacting drugs work. Although dynamic interactions are understandable without silly pictures, here are a couple anyhow.

Dynamic interactions can be **additive/synergistic**, with enhanced effects brought about by combining medications with similar or complementary effects.

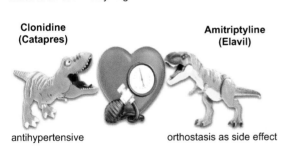

Like-minded "**dyn**os" ganging up to reduce blood pressure, which is an additive/synergistic effect.

Clonidine (Catapres) — antihypertensive

Amitriptyline (Elavil) — orthostasis as side effect

Other dynamic interactions are **antagonistic**, for instance combining a dopaminergic such as pramipexole (for restless legs) with an antidopaminergic like haloperidol (antipsychotic). Here's another example:

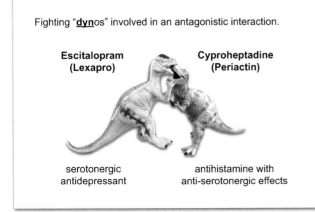

Fighting "**dyn**os" involved in an antagonistic interaction.

Escitalopram (Lexapro) — serotonergic antidepressant

Cyproheptadine (Periactin) — antihistamine with anti-serotonergic effects

PHARMACOKINETIC INTERACTIONS

Kinetics involves the rate at which a drug gets into or out of the body or brain.

Drug-drug Interactions involving absorption are generally straightforward. For instance, anticholinergics slow gut motility and delay gastrointestinal absorption of other medications.

Kinetic interactions involving rate of elimination from the body are challenging to learn and daunting to memorize. It is important to consider these interactions to avoid underdosing or overdosing certain medications. The *Visualize to Memorize* series tackles these tricky elimination interactions by illustrating:

❖ Phase I metabolism involving the six most important cytochrome P450 (CYP450) enzymes **- relevant to most antidepressants**

❖ Phase II metabolism involving UGT enzymes, as applicable to lamotrigine (*Cafer's Mood Stabilizers* book) **- not applicable to antidepressants**

❖ Renal clearance of lithium (*Cafer's Mood Stabilizers* book) **- not applicable to antidepressants**

A mysterious type of kinetic interaction involves drugs getting across the blood-brain barrier, as is necessary for a psychiatric medication to take effect. If such an interaction is occurring, the effect will not be detectable in serum drug levels. This will be discussed in the context of P-glycoprotein (page 9) **- applicable to some antidepressants**

CYTOCHROME P450 ENZYMES

In the liver, kinetic interactions predominantly involve **CYtochrome P450 enzymes**, **CYP** enzymes for short, which can be pronounced "sip". Instead of concerning yourself with the origin of P450 nomenclature, take a moment to contemplate this picture of Ken (kinetic) taking a "sip" (CYP).

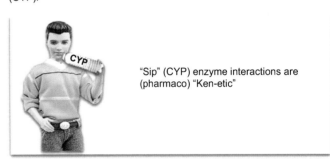

"Sip" (CYP) enzyme interactions are (pharmaco) "Ken-etic"

CYP enzymes, which reside primarily in the liver, make chemicals less lipid-soluble so they can be more easily excreted in urine or bile. Of over 50 CYP enzymes, six play a major role in the biotransformation of medications: 1A2, 2B6, 2C9, 2C19, 2D6 and 3A4. Our visual mnemonics will be built on the following phraseology:

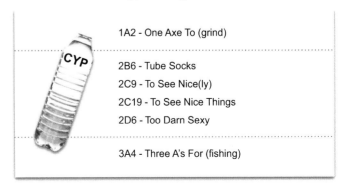

1A2 - One Axe To (grind)

2B6 - Tube Socks
2C9 - To See Nice(ly)
2C19 - To See Nice Things
2D6 - Too Darn Sexy

3A4 - Three A's For (fishing)

The three most important CYPs are **1A2, 2D6** and **3A4**. For psychiatrists, 2C19 can be important, while 2B6 and 2C9 are rarely significant.

SUBSTRATES

A drug that is biotransformed by a particular enzyme is referred to as a **substrate** of that enzyme. When the substrate is biotransformed (metabolized) it is then referred to as a **metabolite**.

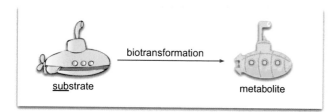

substrate → biotransformation → metabolite

Each CYP enzyme can metabolize several substrates and most substrates can be metabolized by several CYP enzymes. Substrates are the "victims" of the interactions described in this chapter. Throughout this book we use the following visuals for CYP substrates:

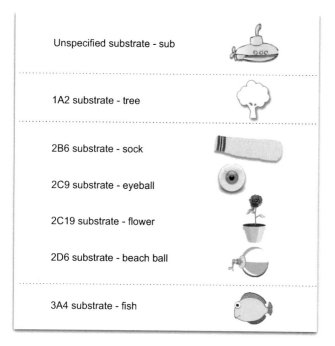

Unspecified substrate - sub

1A2 substrate - tree

2B6 substrate - sock

2C9 substrate - eyeball

2C19 substrate - flower

2D6 substrate - beach ball

3A4 substrate - fish

"Aggressor" medications affect how long victim substrates linger in the blood, and the relative serum concentration of parent drug (substrate) to metabolite. For a given enzyme, interfering medications (aggressors) are either in**D**ucers or in**H**ibitors. **InDucers** stimulate (in**D**uce) production of metabolic enzymes. **InHibitors** interfere with an enzyme's ability to metabolize other medications.

ENZYME IN**H**IBITION

InHibition of an enzyme occurs when one drug (the in**H**ibitor) binds more tightly to the enzyme than the victim substrate binds. The in**H**ibitor itself may be metabolized by the enzyme, or act as a non-competitive inhibitor. When an inhibitor is bound to an enzyme, the victim substrate must find another enzyme to metabolize it, or hope that it can eventually be excreted unchanged. Strong inhibitors may cause the victim substrate to linger longer, prolonging the victim's half-life and elevating its concentration in the blood. For victim substrates that cross the blood brain barrier (as is necessary to be psychoactive), inhibition leads to increased drug concentration in the central nervous system.

Why is **H** being emphasized? Well, when an in**H**ibitor is added to an individual's medication regimen, levels of victim drugs can escalate (**H** for **H**igh). In**H**ibition takes effect quickly, within **H**ours (**H** for **H**urried), although the effect may not be clinically evident for 2 to 4 days, as the victim substrate accumulates.

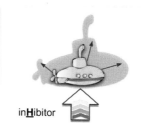

inHibitor

Increased concentration of substrate (and increased ratio of serum substrate:metabolite)

H for **H**igh and **H**urried, within 2–4 hours, although the effect may not be clinically evident for 2–4 days

InHibitors of CYP enzymes will be represented by:

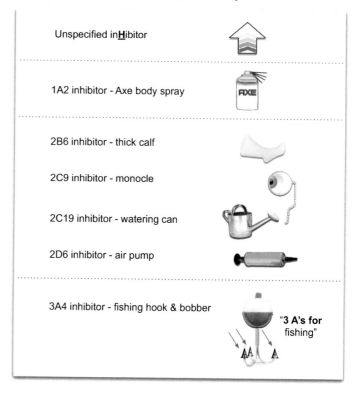

Unspecified inHibitor

1A2 inhibitor - Axe body spray

2B6 inhibitor - thick calf

2C9 inhibitor - monocle

2C19 inhibitor - watering can

2D6 inhibitor - air pump

3A4 inhibitor - fishing hook & bobber

"3 A's for fishing"

Some substrates are also competitive in**H**ibitors of the same CYP enzyme, for instance duloxetine (Cymbalta), which is represented as a both a pump and a beach ball on page 15.

The magnitude to which an in**H**ibitor increases the serum concentration of a specific substrate depends on the number of alternative pathways available to metabolize the substrate. If the drug is a substrate of, e.g., 1A2, 2D6 and 3A4, then inhibiting one of the three pathways should be of no consequence. Such substrates may be described as multi-CYP.

For a substrate metabolized by a single pathway, the effect of inhibition (and induction) will be dramatic. An example is lurasidone (Latuda), which is contraindicated with strong 3A4 inhibitors or inducers.

Some inhibitors are stronger than others. In general, expect blood levels of susceptible substrates to increase in the ballpark of:

❖ mild inhibitor ~ 25% - 50% increase
❖ moderate inhibitor ~ 50% - 100% increase
❖ strong inhibitor > 100% increase

Expect these numbers to vary widely between substrates and individuals, often unpredictably. Note that magnitude of inhibition tends to be dose-related over the dosage range of the inhibitor.

The "**flu**ffers" – notorious strong in**H**ibitors:

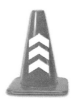

◆ **flu**voxamine (Luvox) - SSRI
◆ **flu**oxetine (Prozac) - SSRI
◆ **flu**conazole (Diflucan) - antifungal
◆ keto**con**azole (Nizoral) - antifungal

The last two are "cone"-azole antifungals.

ENZYME INDUCTION

The opposite of in**H**ibition is in**D**uction. In**D**uction occurs when an in**D**ucer stimulates the liver to produce extra enzymes, leading to enhanced metabolism and quicker clearance of victim drugs.

The **D** is for **D**own, i.e., **D**ecreased serum concentrations of victim substrates. Unlike in**H**ibition (**H** for **H**urried), in**D**uction is **D**elayed, not taking full effect for 2 to 4 weeks while we…
☼ wait for the liver to ramp up enzyme production.

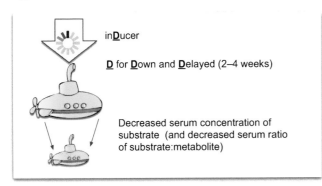

inDucer

D for **D**own and **D**elayed (2–4 weeks)

Decreased serum concentration of substrate (and decreased serum ratio of substrate:metabolite)

InDucers will be depicted by:

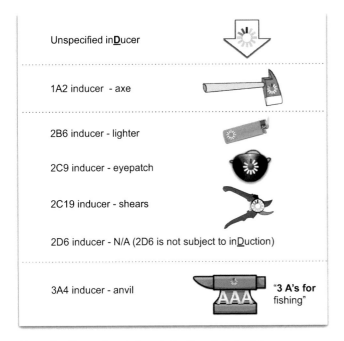

Unspecified inDucer	
1A2 inducer - axe	
2B6 inducer - lighter	
2C9 inducer - eyepatch	
2C19 inducer - shears	
2D6 inducer - N/A (2D6 is not subject to inDuction)	
3A4 inducer - anvil	"3 A's for fishing"

More often than not, an inducer is itself a substrate of the enzyme.

THE SHREDDERS

The **"shredders"** are four **strong inDucers** of several CYPs, which cause countless chemicals to be quickly expelled from the body:

- **carb**amazepine (Tegretol) - antiepileptic
- **pheno**bar**bi**tal (Luminal) - **barbi**turate
- **phenytoin** (Dilantin) - antiepileptic
- **rifampin** (Rifadin) - antimicrobial

Dr. Jonathan Heldt refers to the shredders as **"Carb & Barb"** in his book *Memorable Psychopharmacology*.

St John's Wort (herbal antidepressant) also in**D**uces several CYPs, but does so with less potency than the four shredders.

Can shredding be problematic even if the patient is not taking a victim medication? Consider this:

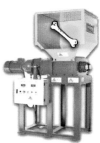

Long-term use of a shredder leads to decreased bone mineral density. This is presumably due to in**D**uction of enzymes that inactivate 25(OH) vitamin **D**.

bone shredding machine

REVERSAL OF INHIBITION/INDUCTION

All things being equal, it is best to avoid prescribing strong inducers or inhibitors. Even if there is no problematic interaction at the time, having a strong inhibitor or inducer on board may complicate future medication management.

Consider an individual on an established medication regimen who stops taking an inducer or inhibitor. The serum concentration of victim substrate(s) will change due to the **reversal** of induction/inhibition.

After an in**D**ucer is withdrawn, the concentration of a victim substrate will increase gradually (**D** for **D**elayed) over a few weeks because the extra CYP enzymes are degraded without being replenished.

When an in**H**ibitor is stopped, levels of a victim substrate will decrease as soon as the aggressor exits the body. "**H**urriedly" does not mean immediately, because it takes about **five half-lives** for the inhibitor to be completely cleared.

For a patient on several psychotropic medications, reversal of inhibition or induction can really throw things out of whack.

 While ePrescribe systems may warn the doctor when starting an interacting medication, there will be **no warning** when stopping a medication will lead to a reversal situation.

For an example of **reversal of in**H**ibition**, consider a patient taking alprazolam (Xanax, 3A4 substrate) who suddenly stops **flu**voxamine (Luvox, 3A4 in**H**ibitor). In absence of the inhibitor, alprazolam levels drop (from double) to normal. Since fluvoxamine has a short elimination half-life of 15 hours, it should be out of the body at 75 hours (15 hr x 5). So, you would expect the patient on Xanax to become more anxious 3 days after stopping Luvox. It may be difficult to discern whether the patient's emerging distress is due to serotonin withdrawal or decreased alprazolam levels.

An example of **reversal of in**D**uction** involves tobacco, which is a 1A2 in**D**ucer. A patient taking clozapine (1A2 substrate) stops smoking, reversing in**D**uction and causing clozapine levels to potentially double over the first week (which is faster than occurs with other inducers). The individual may become obtunded, hypotensive, or even have a seizure. To avoid this, the recommendation is to decrease clozapine dose by 10% daily over the first four days upon smoking cessation, and to check clozapine blood levels before and after the dose adjustment. Note that nicotine products (gum, patches, e-cigs) do not induce 1A2.

Although reversal of in**H**ibition is typically faster than reversal of induction, this does not apply to inhibitors with extremely long half-lives. For instance, **flu**oxetine (Prozac) has a long elimination half-life of about 7 days, keeping itself around for about 35 days (7 days x 5). Consider a patient with schizophrenia on aripiprazole (Abilify, 2D6 substrate) who stops Prozac (2D6 in**H**ibitor). The patient is doing well at one month, but becomes paranoid two months out. Unless the prescriber anticipated this possibility, no one will realize what happened.

PRODRUGS

Phase I metabolism typically involves biotransformation of an active drug to an inactive (or less active) chemical.

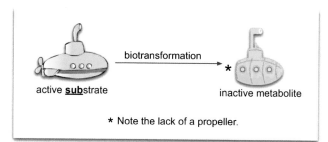

active **sub**strate → biotransformation → inactive metabolite

* Note the lack of a propeller.

For a few medications, the parent drug has low therapeutic activity until it is biotransformed by a CYP enzyme. In such cases, the substrate is called a **prodrug**, and the biotransformation process can be referred to as **bioactivation**.

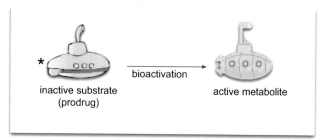

inactive substrate (prodrug) → bioactivation → active metabolite

For most medications (active parent drug to inactive metabolite) in**D**uction decreases (**D** for **D**own) effect of the drug and in**H**ibition (**H** for **H**igh) amplifies the therapeutic effect and/or side effects.

With prodrugs, the opposite effect is observed clinically. Induction increases and inhibition decreases the medication's effect(s).

Don't let prodrugs confuse you. In**H**ibitors increase and in**D**ucers decrease the levels of substrate regardless of whether the parent drug is pharmacologically active.

The following are **prodrugs** activated by 2D6:

❖ **Codeine** - metabolized to morphine
❖ **Tramadol** (Ultram) - weak opioid
❖ **Tamoxifen** - anti-estrogen for breast cancer

The bowling ball is explained on page 15.

PHASE II METABOLISM

Phase II interactions are **not clinically relevant for antidepressants**, but are described here to provide context.

Phase II metabolism occurs in the liver and is subject to kinetic interactions. CYP enzymes are not involved.

Two Kens without a bottle to "CYP" (sip)

Phase II reactions typically involve **conjugation** of a substrate with **glucuronic acid**. This makes the drug water-soluble and prepped for renal excretion.

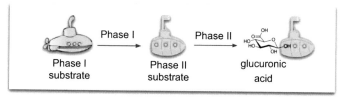

Phase I substrate → Phase I → Phase II substrate → Phase II → glucuronic acid

The responsible enzyme is U̲D̲P̲-g̲lucuronosylt̲ransferase, abbreviated **UGT**, as in "U Got Tagged" with glucuronic acid.

Medications metabolized primarily by Phase II are relatively immune to drug interactions.

RENAL CLEARANCE

A few medications are excreted in urine without being metabolised. Such drugs are not subject to Phase I or II interactions, but may be victims of k̲i̲n̲etic interactions. Renal "aggressors" act by slowing or hastening the rate of excretion of the victim drug in urine.

Interactions affecting renal clearance of victim drugs are also considered (pharmaco)"Ken"etic.

The aggressor in a renal interaction is not referred to as an inducer or inhibitor, because no enzyme is involved. Nor is the victim called a substrate, because it is not being biotransformed.

Lithium, excreted unchanged in urine, is subject to victimization as illustrated in the book *Cafer's Mood Stabilizers and Antiepileptics*.

CYP GENETIC PROFILES

Genetic polymorphisms can influence an individual's medication kinetics, which is most relevant for 2D6 and 2C19. Let's talk about 2D6, arguably the most consequential example. Most antidepressants are 2D6 substrates and some SSRIs are 2C19 substrates.

Most individuals are genetically equipped with 2D6 genes that produce normal 2D6 enzymes that metabolize 2D6 substrates at the usual rate. These normal individuals are said to have a 2D6 **extensive metabolizer** (EM) genotype, resulting in a 2D6 EM phenotype.

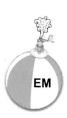

Here is a cute representation of how a normal individual, i.e., 2D6 **extensive metabolizer** (EM), processes 2D6 substrates. The air inside the beach ball represents the substrate, which is being expelled from the ball as metabolite at the usual rate. 2D6 substrates will have typical elimination half-lives.

About 5% of the population have extra copies of 2D6 genes, resulting in an **ultrarapid metabolizer** (UM) phenotype. These individuals clear 2D6 substrates quickly.

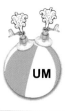

For 2D6 **ultrarapid metabolizers** (UM), the air (2D6 substrate) flows out of the ball quickly as metabolite. 2D6 substrates could be ineffective for these individuals (with the exception of 2D6 prodrugs, which could be be too strong).

About 10% of individuals have defective 2D6 enzymes resulting in a 2D6 **poor metabolizer** (PM) phenotype. This condition may be found on a diagnosis list as "Cytochrome P450 2D6 enzyme deficiency".

For 2D6 "**POOR ME**"tabolizers (PM), air accumulates, resulting in unexpectedly long half-lives for 2D6 substrates. These individuals are more likely to report side effects.

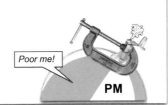

Poor me!

PM

An individual taking a strong 2D6 in**H**ibitor (pump as illustrated on page 15) will metabolize 2D6 substrates **as if** the individual had a 2D6 PM genotype.

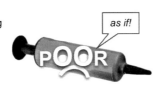

as if!

POOR

In summary, genetic testing of CYP polymorphisms will interpret the individual's metabolizer profile for a given enzyme as either:

❖ Extensive metabolizer (EM) - normal
❖ Ultrarapid metabolizer (UM) - fast clearance of substrates
❖ Poor metabolizer (PM) - slow clearance of substrates

A genetic test result of **intermediate metabolizer** (IM) means that enzyme activity is likely to be a bit lower than that of an EM, i.e., an intermediate between EM and PM. Generally, IM individuals can be clinically managed normally, like an EM individual.

Standalone 2D6 genotyping costs at least $200. GeneSight or Genecept panels cost about $4,000 and report the six relevant CYPs and two UGT enzymes (UGT1A4 and UGT2B15). 23andMe ($199) reports 1A2, 2C9, and 2C19, among 100s of other genes. 23andMe does not report the most relevant CYP genotype, 2D6, because the genetics of 2D6 metabolism is more complicated.

Genotyping may be useful when choosing which medication to prescribe an individual patient. With GeneSight, about 1 in 5 patients have a genetic variation relevant to their treatment. For an individual already established on a medication, serum drug levels may be more useful than genotyping.

Therapeutic serum ranges are defined for three tricyclic antidepressants (TCAs): desipramine, imipramine and nortriptyline —"mosquitos DINe on your blood".

P-GLYCOPROTEIN

P-glycoprotein (P-gp) is a gatekeeper at the gut lumen and the blood-brain barrier. P-gp pumps P-gp substrates out of the brain—"Pumpers gonna pump". Sertraline (Zoloft) and paroxetine (Paxil) are two antidepressants shown to inhibit P-gp.

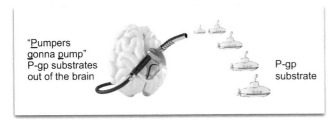

"Pumpers gonna pump" P-gp substrates out of the brain

P-gp substrate

An example of a relevant P-gp interaction involves the OTC opioid antidiarrheal loperamide (Imodium). Loperamide does not cause central opioid effects under normal circumstances. If the individual takes a potent P-gp inhibitor, megadose loperamide can stay in the brain long enough to cause euphoria.

THE NATURE OF THIS INFORMATION

The information presented in the remainder of this chapter is a synthesis of sources including the OpeRational ClassificAtion (ORCA) system (as presented in *The Top 100 Drug Interactions* by Hansten & Horn, 2019), Lexicomp, DrugBank, Flockhart Table, ePocrates, Carlat Medication Fact Book, Stahl's Essential Psychopharmacology, The Medical Letter, Current Psychiatry, GeneSight, Genecept, various research papers and FDA prescribing information for the individual drugs.

Reputable sources are often at odds with each other regarding the strength of specific inducers/inhibitors, the vulnerability of specific substrates to induction/inhibition, or even which CYPs are relevant to a specific medication. CYP interactions are continuously being discovered and clarified. Even with the freshest information and full knowledge of a patient's genotype, the magnitude of a specific CYP interaction is difficult to predict.

HOW TO APPLY THIS INFORMATION

Refer to the tables on pages 19 and 20. Medications featured in this book are highlighted for you. First acquaint yourself with the in**D**ucers because the list is short. Memorize the bolded inducers (shredders). After you know the inducers, move to the in**H**ibitor column. Memorize the bolded inhibitors (fluffers) and your highlighted medications.

When it comes to substrates, memorization is less important. Substrates are only relevant when an inducer or inhibitor is on board, or if the patient has a special metabolizer genotype. Of the medications you prescribe, be aware of the more susceptible substrates.

Consider running an interaction check whenever a patient is taking a shredder, fluffer, systemic antifungal, HIV medication, or cancer medication. ePocrates.com and the ePocrates app are adequate, and free.

Keep things simple. When choosing new medications, avoid major inducers and inhibitors if suitable alternatives are available. For the complicated psychiatric patient on several medications, try to avoid carbamazepine (shredder inducer) and the **flu**ffer SSRIs (**flu**oxetine and **flu**voxamine). Among SSRIs, escitalopram (Lexapro) and sertraline (Zoloft) are good choices—they are 2C19 substrates but do not affect the metabolism of other medications.

Also think about choosing less vulnerable substrates. Each drug mascot on pages 17 and 18 is depicted in box/bubble because it is generally not involved in clinically significant kinetic interactions (although dynamic interactions almost always apply). You don't have to worry much about benzodiazepine interactions if you stick to the "LOT" benzos—**l**orazepam, **o**xazepam and **t**emazepam. Most antipsychotics are susceptible substrates, but not so much for ziprasidone, loxapine and paliperidone.

This book uses picture association as a memorization technique. Pages 10 through 16 establish a visual mnemonic framework for various kinetic interactions that will be reinforced by a mascot for each medication. The mascots serve a double purpose of helping you remember US trade name/generic name pairings.

Since you probably won't be mentioning CYP nomenclature in casual conversation, you might want to bypass the technical naming system altogether. Instead of keeping a list of "3A4 substrates" in your memory bank, you could just learn the school of "fish".

I hope this book empowers you to understand and memorize topics that are otherwise daunting, so you can to use your knowledge to improve patient care. Without further ado, let's start our journey to becoming a superhero of psychotropic medication management.

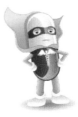

Cytochrome P450 1A2 (CYP1A2)
"One Axe to Grind; One Axe to Grow"

1A2 accounts for 10–15% of CYP activity in the liver

52% of individuals are 1A2 ultrarapid metabolizers; < 1% are poor metabolizers

"**1** **A**xe to **2** Grind"

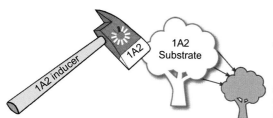

in**D**ucer = **D**own

Decreased substrate levels

induction onsets and reverses slowly = **D**elayed *

Hydrocarbons from smoked herbs such as tobacco and cannabis are moderate potency 1A2 inducers. All other 1A2 inducers are weak.

"**1** **A**xe **2** Grow"

in**H**ibitor = **H**igh

Increased substrate levels

in**H**ibition happens within **H**ours = **H**urried and reverses as soon as the inhibitor is cleared from the body (five half-lives of the inhibitor)

Fluvoxamine (Luvox) is the only strong 1A2 inhibitor.

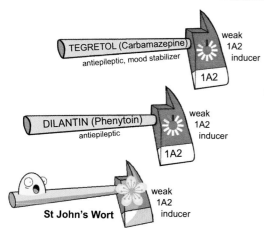

TEGRETOL (Carbamazepine) — antiepileptic, mood stabilizer — weak 1A2 inducer

DILANTIN (Phenytoin) — antiepileptic — weak 1A2 inducer

St John's Wort — weak 1A2 inducer

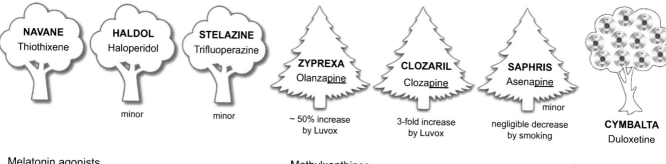

Tobacco — cannabis also — moderate inducer — **not** nicotine patch or gum

* Induction by smoking takes about 3 days to start—notice the axe has no spinning wheel like the other axes. Upon cessation of smoking, induction reverses over the first week. This is much faster than with other inducers. 10 cigarettes daily is sufficient for maximum induction effect.

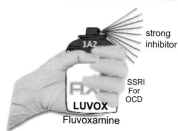

LUVOX — Fluvoxamine — strong inhibitor — SSRI For OCD

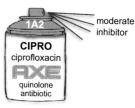

CIPRO — ciprofloxacin — quinolone antibiotic — moderate inhibitor

First Generation Antipsychotics

NAVANE Thiothixene

HALDOL Haloperidol — minor

STELAZINE Trifluoperazine — minor

Second Generation Antipsychotics "-pine" trees

ZYPREXA Olanza**pine** — ~ 50% increase by Luvox

CLOZARIL Cloza**pine** — 3-fold increase by Luvox

SAPHRIS Asena**pine** — minor — negligible decrease by smoking

Antidepressant

CYMBALTA Duloxetine

Melatonin agonists

* **ROZEREM** Ramelteon — up to 100-fold increase by Luvox

HETLIOZ Tasimelteon

Melatonin

Methylxanthines

Theophylline — "TREE -ophylline" — 3-fold increase by Luvox

Caffeine

NOURIANZ Istradefylline

Spasmolytic

** **ZANAFLEX** Tizanidine — > 10-fold increase by Luvox

* Contraindicated with Luvox
** Contraindicated with Luvox or Cipro

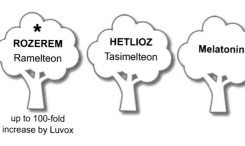

Tobacco — Clozapine or Olanzapine — 50%

Tobacco **D**ecreases blood levels of these two "pine trees" by about 50%.

Conclusion: Keep in mind that 52% of individuals have a 1A2 ultrarapid metabolizer genotype, and everyone who smokes has an ultrarapid metabolizer phenotype. Smokers may need to take higher doses of 1A2 substrates. The effect of smoking on olanzapine and clozapine is worthy of memorization. Memorization of other 1A2 substrates is of lower priority, as long as you remember to run an interaction check on any medication regimen that includes Luvox. Consider keeping Luvox out of the mix entirely—it is nonessential for treatment of OCD because other SSRIs are equally effective at high doses (page 34).

Ciprofloxacin, a moderate 1A2 in**H**ibitor, increases clozapine levels about 2-fold.

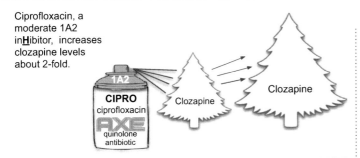

Fluvoxamine, a strong 1A2 in**H**ibitor ("**Flu**ffer") increases clozapine levels 3-fold on average, but up to 10-fold in some cases.

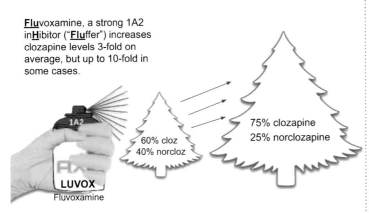

60% cloz 40% norcloz

75% clozapine 25% norclozapine

Kinetic interactions can be more complicated than simply increasing/decreasing concentrations of victim substrates.

Combining clozapine and fluvoxamine is hazardous, but can potentially be used for therapeutic advantage. Close monitoring of serum **clozapine levels** would be required.

Norclozapine is the main metabolite of clozapine, formed by 1A2 metabolism. When clozapine blood levels are reported, clozapine and metabolite (norclozapine) levels are provided separately. Through 1A2 in**H**ibition, Luvox increases the serum **clozapine:norclozapine ratio**. A **H**igher serum clozapine:norclozapine ratio is generally considered desirable*. Norclozapine provides little antipsychotic benefit and causes weight gain, diabetes, seizures, and neutropenia.

Patients given clozapine 100 mg + Luvox 50 mg daily (compared to clozapine 300 mg monotherapy) demonstrated more improvement with less weight gain and less drooling. Clozapine levels were similar for both groups with, as expected, lower norclozapine levels for those taking Luvox.
(Lu ML et al, 2018; randomized controlled trial, N=85).

*The negative aspect of a **H**igher clozapine:norclozapine is greater anticholinergic burden. Clozapine is anticholinergic, whereas norclozapine is cholinergic. Consequently, clozapine causes constipation, while norclozapine does not. The anticholinergic properties of clozapine may impair cognition, whereas norclozapine may provide cognitive benefits such as enhanced working memory.

Certain physiologic states may increase levels of olanzapine and clozapine up to 2-fold.

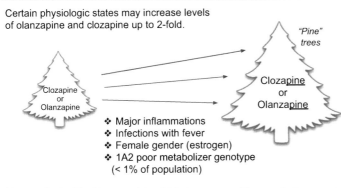

"Pine" trees

Clozapine or Olanzapine

❖ Major inflammations
❖ Infections with fever
❖ Female gender (estrogen)
❖ 1A2 poor metabolizer genotype (< 1% of population)

For a patient with efficacy or tolerability issues, consider monitoring serum levels of the antipsychotic. The author checks clozapine levels routinely, and olanzapine levels in some cases.

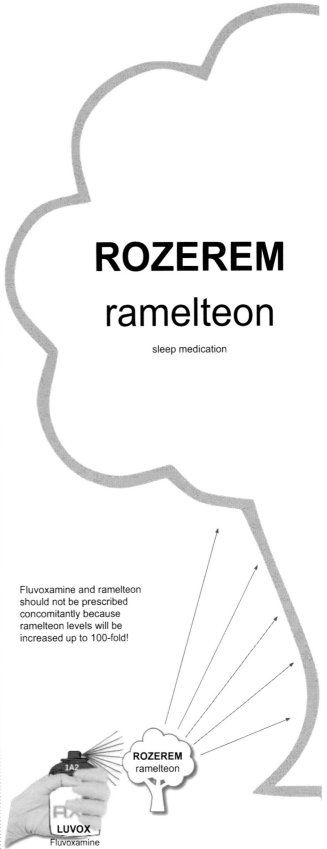

ROZEREM
ramelteon
sleep medication

Fluvoxamine and ramelteon should not be prescribed concomitantly because ramelteon levels will be increased up to 100-fold!

Cytochrome P450 2B6 (CYP2B6)
"Tube Socks"

3% of individuals are 2B6 ultrarapid metabolizers; 7% are poor metabolizers

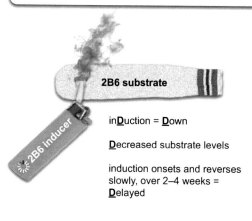

inDuction = Down

Decreased substrate levels

induction onsets and reverses slowly, over 2–4 weeks = Delayed

There are no strong 2B6 inducers.

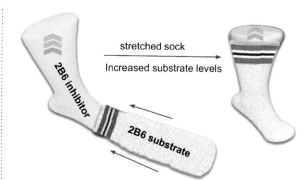

stretched sock
Increased substrate levels

inHibition = High

inHibition happens within Hours = Hurried and reverses as soon as the inhibitor is cleared from the body (five half-lives of the inhibitor)

There are no strong 2B6 inhibitors.

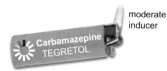
moderate inducer

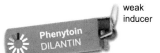
weak inducer

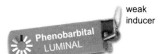
weak inducer

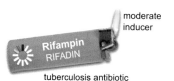
moderate inducer

tuberculosis antibiotic

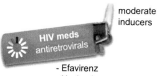
moderate inducers

- Efavirenz
- Nevirapine
- Ritonavir

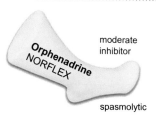
moderate inhibitor

spasmolytic

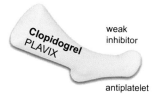
weak inhibitor

antiplatelet

Opioid
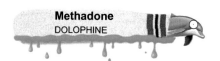

Alkylating Drugs for Cancer

Cyclophosphamide
CYTOXAN

Ifosfamide
IFEX

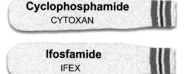

NNRTIs for HIV

Efavirenz
SUSTIVA

Nevirapine
VIRAMUNE

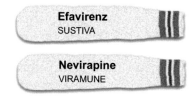

Anaesthetic

Propofol
DIPRIVAN

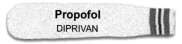

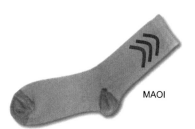
MAOI

Selegiline
ELDEPRYL, EMSAM

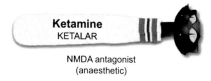

Ketamine
KETALAR

NMDA antagonist (anaesthetic)

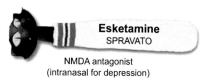

Esketamine
SPRAVATO

NMDA antagonist (intranasal for depression)

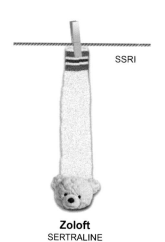
SSRI

Zoloft
SERTRALINE

NDRI antidepressant
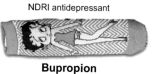

Bupropion
WELLBUTRIN

Conclusion: Fortunately, there are no strong inhibitors or inducers of 2B6. For psychiatrists, 2B6 is of minimal significance, unless methadone is being prescribed. You will want to run an interaction check (e.g., ePocrates or Lexicomp) whenever a medication regimen includes a shredder, cancer medication, HIV medication, or systemic antifungal.

For psychiatry, 2C9 interactions are of little clinical significance. Paroxetine (Paxil) is the only antidepressant on this page.

Cytochrome P450 2C9 (CYP2C9)
"To See Nice(ly)"

0% of individuals are 2C9 ultrarapid metabolizers; 5% are poor metabolizers

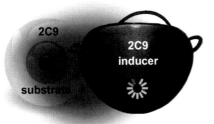

inDuction = Down

Decreased substrate levels

induction onsets and reverses slowly, over 2–4 weeks = Delayed

There are no strong 2C9 inducers.

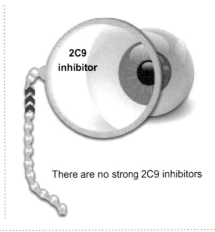

inHibition = High

Increased substrate levels

inHibition happens within Hours = Hurried

Inhibition reverses as soon as the inhibitor is cleared from the body (five half-lives of the inhibitor)

There are no strong 2C9 inhibitors

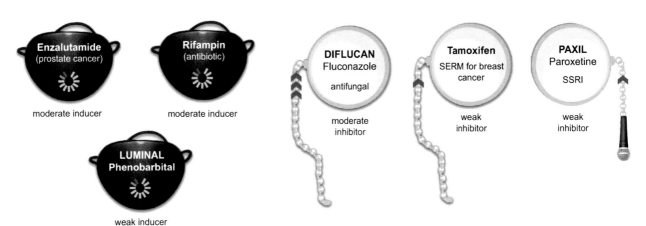

Enzalutamide (prostate cancer) — moderate inducer

Rifampin (antibiotic) — moderate inducer

LUMINAL Phenobarbital — weak inducer

DIFLUCAN Fluconazole — antifungal — moderate inhibitor

Tamoxifen SERM for breast cancer — weak inhibitor

PAXIL Paroxetine — SSRI — weak inhibitor

Antiepileptics

DILANTIN
Phenytoin

"d-EYE-lantin; phen-EYE-toin"

Also 2C19

DEPAKOTE
Valproate

"Dep-EYE-kote"

2C9 contributes only 25% to the metabolism of VPA

Anticoagulant

COUMADIN
Warfarin

"coum-EYE-din"

Also 2C19

Sulfonylureas for DM

MICRONASE
Glyburide

"glybur-EYED"

AMARYL
Glimepiride

"glimepir-EYED"

GLUCOTROL
Glipizide

"Glipiz-EYED"

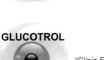

ORINASE
Tolbutamide

"tolbutam-EYED"

ARB for HTN

COZAAR
Losartan

"Coz-EYEr"

Also 3A4

Lipid lowering

LESCOL
Fluvastatin

"fluv-EYE-statin"

Libido enhancer

ADDYI
Flibanserin

"Add-EYE"

NSAID

FELDENE
Piroxicam

"p-EYE-roxicam"

COX-2 inhibitor

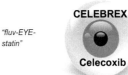

CELEBREX
Celecoxib

"cel-EYE-brex"

Conclusion: Consider checking valproic acid (VPA) levels more often if the patient is taking or stops taking enzalutamide, rifampin, or diflucan; but don't expect much variance from baseline. Consider avoiding paroxetine entirely (page 44).

Cytochrome P450 2C19 (CYP2C19)
"To See Nice Things (grow)"

10% of individuals are 2C19 ultrarapid metabolizers; 5% are poor metabolizers

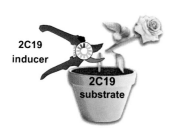

2C19 inducer

inDuction = Down

Decreased substrate levels

induction onsets and reverses slowly, over 2–4 weeks = Delayed

2C19 substrate

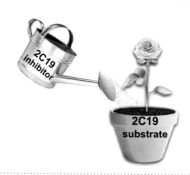

inHibition = High

Increased substrate levels

inHibition happens within Hours = Hurried

Inhibition reverses as soon as the inhibitor is cleared from the body (five half-lives of the inhibitor)

2C19 substrate

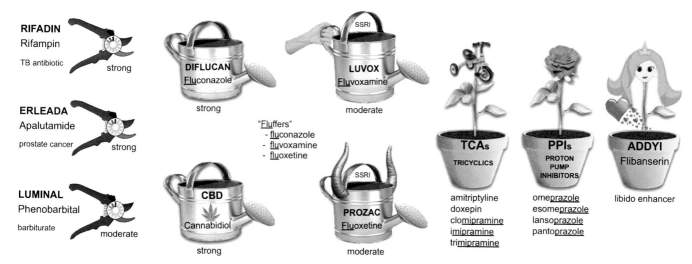

RIFADIN
Rifampin
TB antibiotic — strong

ERLEADA
Apalutamide
prostate cancer — strong

LUMINAL
Phenobarbital
barbiturate — moderate

DIFLUCAN
Fluconazole
strong

CBD
Cannabidiol
strong

LUVOX
Fluvoxamine
moderate

PROZAC
Fluoxetine
moderate

"Fluffers"
- fluconazole
- fluvoxamine
- fluoxetine

TCAs
TRICYCLICS
amitriptyline
doxepin
clomipramine
imipramine
trimipramine

PPIs
PROTON PUMP INHIBITORS
omeprazole
esomeprazole
lansoprazole
pantoprazole

ADDYI
Flibanserin
libido enhancer

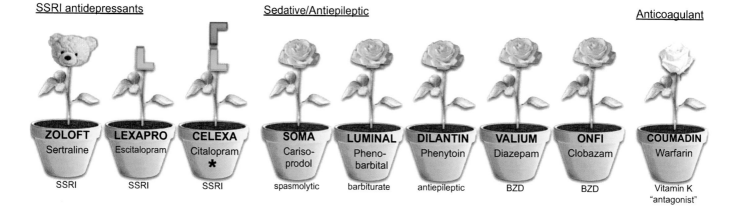

SSRI antidepressants

ZOLOFT
Sertraline
SSRI

LEXAPRO
Escitalopram
SSRI

CELEXA
Citalopram
*
SSRI

Sedative/Antiepileptic

SOMA
Cariso-prodol
spasmolytic

LUMINAL
Pheno-barbital
barbiturate

DILANTIN
Phenytoin
antiepileptic

VALIUM
Diazepam
BZD

ONFI
Clobazam
BZD

Anticoagulant

COUMADIN
Warfarin
Vitamin K "antagonist"

2C19 poor metabolizers (PM)

Individuals with a 2C19 PM genotype clear 2C19 substrates slowly, leading to Higher blood levels (as if they were taking a 2C19 inHibitor). Standard doses of 2C19 substrates may be too strong.

* 2C19 poor metabolizers should not exceed 20 mg of citalopram (QT prolongation).

5% of population (20% of Asians)

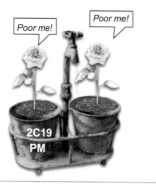

Poor me! *Poor me!*

2C19 PM

2C19 ultrarapid metabolizers (UM)

2C19 UM individuals clear 2C19 substrates quickly, leading to low blood levels. These individuals are more likely to be non-responders to 2C19 substrates at standard doses.

10% of population

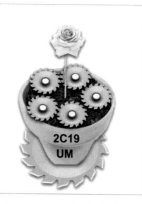

2C19 UM

Conclusion: 2C19 genotyping is not typically ordered as a standalone test, but if 2C19 metabolizer genotype is known (e.g., from GeneSight or Genecept), the information can be put to good use when dosing (es)citalopram and sertraline. Knowledge of metabolizer status is not essential because these SSRIs can be titrated the old-fashioned way, according to response and side effects. In any event, avoid prescribing Soma, Valium, or phenobarbital for anxiety due to their particularly high risk of abuse and dependence. Avoid St. John's Wort due to interactions, and because it only works for mild depression.

Cytochrome P450 2D6 (CYP2D6)
"Too Darn Sexy"

2D6 metabolizes ~ 12% of prescription drugs. Notice how all of the -oxetine's are 2D6 inhibitors and/or substrates.

5% of individuals are 2D6 ultrarapid metabolizers (UM).
10% are poor metabolizers (PM).

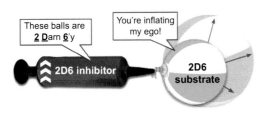

These balls are 2 **D**arn **6**'y

You're inflating my ego!

inHibition = High

Increased substrate levels

inHibition happens within Hours = Hurried

Inhibition reverses as soon as the inhibitor is cleared from the body (five half-lives of the inhibitor)

2D6 enzymes cannot be induced.

Prodrugs are substrates that are less potent than their metabolites. Ordinary substrates (beach balls) are deactivated by 2D6. Prodrugs (bowling balls) are *activated* by 2D6. In the presence of an inhibitor prodrugs are less effective.

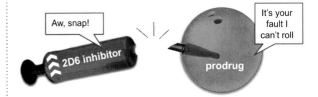

Aw, snap!

It's your fault I can't roll

prodrug

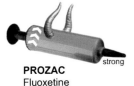

PROZAC
Fluoxetine — strong

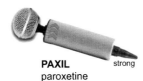

PAXIL
paroxetine — strong

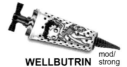

WELLBUTRIN
Bupropion — mod/strong

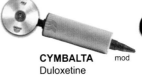

CYMBALTA
Duloxetine — mod

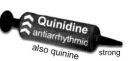

Quinidine antiarrhythmic
also quinine — strong

Antidepressants

SPARI

TRINTELLIX
vortioxetine

SNRI

CYMBALTA
duloxetine
"Cym-BALL-ta"

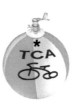
OH-bup-ropion

OH-bupropion
active metabolite of bupropion (Wellbutrin)

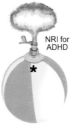

Tricyclic antidepressants

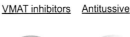
NRI for ADHD

STRATTERA
atomoxetine

VMAT inhibitors

AUSTEDO
deutetra-benazine
also tetrabenazine

Antitussive

dextro-methorphan

Anti-HTN

LOPRESSOR
metoprolol
beta blocker

First Generation Antipsychotics (FGA)

*
HALDOL
haloperidol

**
TRILAFON
perphenazine

**
MELLARIL
thioridazine

**
ORAP
pimozide
2D6 genotyping required

Second Generation Antipsychotics (SGA)

(*)
ABILIFY
aripiprazole
also 3A4 substrate

*
FANAPT
iloperidone

*
REXULTI
brexpiprazole

Prodrugs

Codeine
metabolized to morphine

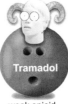
Tramadol
weak opioid and SNRI

Tamoxifen
breast cancer

2D6 poor metabolizers have defective 2D6 enzymes. Substrates are cleared slowly (by other pathways) or are unmetabolized leading to Higher blood levels, **as if** the patient were taking an inHibitor.

POOR — as if !

** 2D6 genotyping is recommended prior to starting these medications, which are increased 3--4-fold in 2D6 PMs. Mellaril is contraindicated for 2D6 PMs.

* 50% dose reduction is recommended for 2D6 poor metabolizers.

(*) According to the label, use 75% of Abilify dose if the individual is a 2D6 PM. Use 50% Abilify dose if 2D6 PM and taking a 3A4 inhibitor.

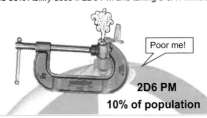

Poor me!

2D6 PM
10% of population

2D6 extensive metabolizers
have the typical genotype and process 2D6 substrates as expected

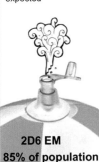

2D6 EM
85% of population

2D6 ultrarapid metabolizers
clear 2D6 substrates quickly. These individuals are more likely to be non-responders to 2D6 substrates (excluding 2D6 prodrugs, which may be too strong). This genotype is relatively common among those with Middle Eastern or North African heritage.

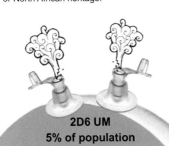

2D6 UM
5% of population

Conclusion: 2D6 interactions need to be understood by prescribers of antidepressants and antipsychotics. To avoid 2D6 interactions, use Lexapro or Zoloft instead of Prozac/Paxil.

Among the CYP genetic assays, 2D6 is the most useful. The test is about $200 as a standalone, and is recommended prior to starting Trilafon, Mellaril, or Orap—three antipsychotics that psychiatrists rarely prescribe. For the other 2D6 substrates, serum drug levels may be more useful than genotyping. The author checks blood levels of haloperidol, risperidone and aripiprazole when there are issues with efficacy or tolerability.

Cytochrome P450 3A4 (CYP3A4)
"3 A's For (fishing)"

> 50% of prescription drugs are 3A4 substrates—plenty of fish!

0% of individuals are 3A4 ultrarapid metabolizers; < 1% are poor metabolizers

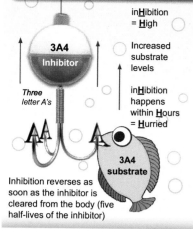

inHibition = High

Increased substrate levels

inHibition happens within Hours = Hurried

3A4 Inhibitor

Three letter A's

3A4 substrate

Inhibition reverses as soon as the inhibitor is cleared from the body (five half-lives of the inhibitor)

inDuction = Down

Decreased substrate levels

induction onsets and reverses slowly, over 2–4 weeks = **D**elayed

3A4 AAA inducer

3A4 substrate

Macrolide Antibiotics (-mycins)

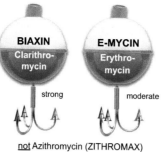

BIAXIN Clarithro-mycin — strong

E-MYCIN Erythro-mycin — moderate

not Azithromycin (ZITHROMAX)

Systemic Antifungals (-conazoles)

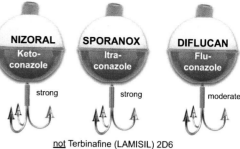

NIZORAL Keto-conazole — strong

SPORANOX Itra-conazole — strong

DIFLUCAN Flu-conazole — moderate

not Terbinafine (LAMISIL) 2D6

Antidepressant

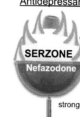

Grapefruit Juice — moderate

SERZONE Nefazodone — strong

HIV meds (-avirs)

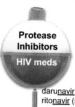

Protease Inhibitors HIV meds

darunavir (mod)
ritonavir (strong)
atazanavir (strong)
etc

Calcium Channel Blockers

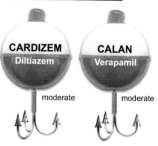

CARDIZEM Diltiazem — moderate

CALAN Verapamil — moderate

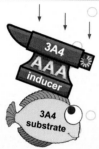

* PDE-5 inhibitors — Viagra, etc

** ADDYI Flibanserin

Contra-ceptives — Estrogens, progestins

* VIIBRYD Vilazodone

* INGREZZA Valbenazine

SUBOXONE Buprenorphine

** DAYVIGO Lemborexant
also suvorexant (Belsomra), to a lesser extent

* BUSPAR Buspirone

There is risk of rhabdomyolysis when HMG-CoA reductase inhibitors (statins) are combined with 3A4 inHibitors.

** STATINS — simvastatin, atorvastatin

not:
Pravastatin (Pravachol)
Rosuvastatin (Crestor)
Fluvastatin (Lescol)

Benzodiazepines

** XANAX Alprazolam

LIBRIUM Chlordiazepoxide

KLONOPIN Clonazepam

also:
Diazepam (Valium)
Estazolam (Prosom) **
Midazolam (Versed) **
Triazolam (Halcion) **
Clorazepate (Tranxene)

not:
Lorazepam (Ativan)
Oxazepam (Serax)
Temazepam (Restoril)
Clobazam (Onfi) 2C19

Antipsychotics

** LATUDA Lurasidone

Lurasidone is metabolized exclusively by 3A4 and is contraindicated with potent 3A4 inhibitors or inducers.

* SEROQUEL Quetiapine

Quetiapine levels are increased 6-fold by strong 3A4 inhibitors and decreased 6-fold by strong inducers.

* ABILIFY Aripiprazole — also 2D6

** CAPLYTA Lumateperone

* REXULTI Brexpiprazole

* VRAYLAR Cariprazine

** ORAP Pimozide — also 2D6

* NUPLAZID Pimavanserin

minor 3A4 substrates:
Chlorpromazine (Thorazine)
Clozapine (Clozaril)
Haloperidol (Haldol)
Iloperidone (Fanapt)
Loxapine (Loxitane)
Prochlorperazine
Perphenazine (Trilafon)
Risperidone (Risperdal)
Ziprasidone (Geodon)

not:
Asenapine (Saphris) 1A2
Fluphenazine (Prolixin) 2D6
Molindone (Moban)
Olanzapine (Zyprexa) 1A2
Paliperidone (Invega)
Promethazine (Phenergan)
Thiothixene (Navane) 1A2
Trifluoperazine (Stelazine) 1A2

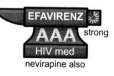

DILANTIN AAA Phenytoin — strong

TEGRETOL AAA Carbamazepine — strong

LUMINAL AAA Phenobarbital — strong
primidone also

RIFAMPIN AAA antibiotic — strong

EFAVIRENZ AAA HIV med — strong
nevirapine also

St John's Wort — mod

PROVIGIL AAA Modafinil — mod

weaker: Nuvigil (armodafinil)

* Dosing adjustments defined

** Has contraindications related to kinetic interactions

Conclusion: 3A4 is the workhorse of CYP metabolism, accounting for 30% of hepatic CYP activity and 70% of CYP activity in the gut. Since > 50% of drugs are 3A4 substrates, think twice before prescribing strong 3A4 inhibitors or inducers.

Non-participants

Medications that do not become significantly involved in <u>kinetic</u> interactions are depicted **"in a bubble"**.

Some of these medications are **"in a box"** (with a hole in it) to indicate that kinetic interactions exist, but usually do not need be taken into consideration when prescribing the medication.

<u>Dynamic</u> interactions still apply to bubbled/boxed medications.

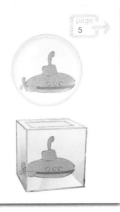

page 5 →

We will display medications "in a bubble" or "in a box" if they are not expected to serve as *clinically significant* substrates, inducers or inhibitors. There is a hole at the top of the boxes to suggest some degree of vulnerability to relevant kinetic interactions, but not to an extent prescribers need to routinely worry about. In general, medications that are renally cleared have relatively few drug–drug interactions because their metabolism does not rely on CYP enzymes.

For a substrate metabolized through multiple pathways, serum levels are not significantly affected by in**H**ibition of a single CYP. For instance, over half of prescription drugs are 3A4 substrates, but will not be depicted as fish (page 16) if they are multi-CYP substrates. Multi-CYP substrates are depicted in a box (not a bubble) because interactions do occur but are unlikely to matter much.

A multi-CYP substrate is more likely to be victimized by an in**D**ucer than by an in**H**ibitor. It is worthwhile to run an interaction check on a patient's medication list if they are taking a "shredder" in**D**ucer (page 7), even for the boxed medications.

A bubble/box certifies the medication is:
* No more than a weak CYP inducer or inducer, and...
* Either a multi-CYP substrate or a substrate not metabolized by any CYP

A bubble does **not** imply that a medication does not participate in <u>dynamic</u> interactions, because almost all drugs do. Acamprosate (Campral) and N-acetylcysteine (NAC) are rare exceptions, depicted in a double bubble.

This book contains medication monographs with mascots designed to help you pair antidepressant trade names with generic names, and remember kinetic interactions. Medications featured in this book are highlighted. Refer to *Cafer's Psychopharmacology* for all of the mascots, 270 in total.

Dynamic interactions:
Not applicable to every drug in class

"Bubbled" or "boxed" medications are unlikely to be involved in clinically significant <u>kinetic</u> interactions:

Antipsychotics

* Extrapyramidal effects
* Sedation
* Weight gain
* Hyperglycemia
* QT prolongation
* Myelosuppression
* Anticholinergic
* Proconvulsant

INVEGA
Paliperidone

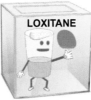
GEODON
Ziprasidone

LOXITANE
Loxapine

MOBAN
Molindone

COMPAZINE
Prochlorperazine

Antidepressants

* Serotonergic
* QT prolongation
* Sedation
* Weight gain
* Hyponatremia
* Antiplatelet
* Hypo/hypertension
* Anticholinergic

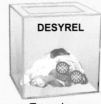
DESYREL
Trazodone

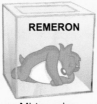
REMERON
Mirtazapine

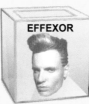
EFFEXOR
Venlafaxine

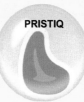
PRISTIQ
Desvenlafaxine

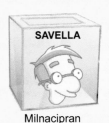
SAVELLA
Milnacipran

Antiepileptics

* Sedation
* Stevens-Johnson Syndrome
* Hyponatremia
* Acidosis
* Myelosuppression

NEURONTIN
Gabapentin

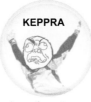
KEPPRA
Levetiracetam

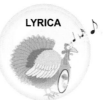
LYRICA
Pregabalin

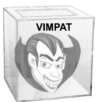
VIMPAT
Lacosamide

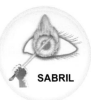
SABRIL
Vigabatrin

Sedatives

* Sedation
* Respiratory depression

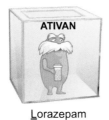
ATIVAN
<u>L</u>orazepam

SERAX
<u>O</u>xazepam

RESTORIL
<u>T</u>emazepam

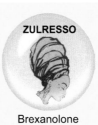
ZULRESSO
Brexanolone

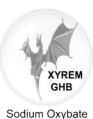
XYREM GHB
Sodium Oxybate

The 3 "<u>LOT</u>" benzos—No CYP interactions but levels may double with VPA (Depakote) due to UGT2B15 in**H**ibition

Dynamic interactions:
Not applicable to every drug in class

"Bubbled" or "boxed" medications are unlikely to be involved in clinically significant <u>kinetic</u> interactions:

Antihistamines

- ❖ Anticholinergic
  - constipation
  - urinary retention
  - cognitive impairment
- ❖ Sedation

BENADRYL
Diphenhydramine

UNISOM
Doxylamine

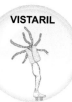
VISTARIL
Hydroxyzine

ANTIVERT
Meclizine

antiserotonergic
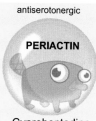
PERIACTIN
Cyproheptadine

Anticholinergics

- ❖ Anticholinergic
  - constipation
  - urinary retention
  - cognitive impairment
- ❖ Sedation

COGENTIN
Benztropine

ARTANE
Trihexyphenidyl

SYMMETREL
Amantadine

BENTYL
Dicyclomine

ROBINUL
Glycopyrrolate

Cognitive Enhancers

- ❖ Cholinergic
- ❖ Lowers seizure threshold

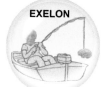
EXELON
Rivastigmine

RAZADYNE
Galantamine

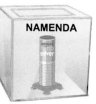
NAMENDA
Memantine

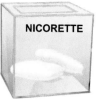
NICORETTE
Nicotine

The hydrocarbons in smoked tobacco in**D**uce 1A2. Nicotine itself does not.

Addiction Medicine

For some, dynamic interactions are part of their mechanism of action, e.g., opioid antagonism by naltrexone and naloxone.

CHANTIX
Varenicline

ReVIA
Naltrexone

NARCAN
Naloxone

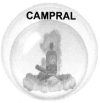
CAMPRAL
Acamprosate

Double bubble: acamprosate has no known kinetic or dynamic interactions.

Sympatholytics

- ❖ Hypotension
- ❖ Bradycardia
- ❖ Sedation / fatigue

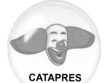
CATAPRES
Clonidine

MINIPRESS
Prazosin

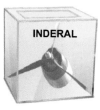
INDERAL
Propranolol

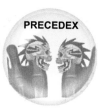
PRECEDEX
Dexmedetomidine

Spasmolytics

- ❖ Sedative
- ❖ Hypotensive
- ❖ Anticholinergics
- ❖ Lowers seizure threshold

ROBAXIN
Methocarbamol

LIORESAL
Baclofen

serotonergic
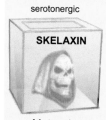
SKELAXIN
Metaxalone

Stimulants

- ❖ Hypertensive
- ❖ Dopaminergic
- ❖ Noradrenergic
- ❖ Lowers seizure threshold

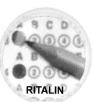
RITALIN
Methylphenidate

SUNOSI
Solriamfetol

Supplements

Double bubble: NAC has no known kinetic or dynamic interactions.

NAC
N-acetylcysteine

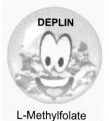
DEPLIN
L-Methylfolate

RELEVANT PHARMACOKINETIC INTERACTIONS, general overview with included medications highlighted

INDUCERS
InDuction Decreases substrates slowly, over 2 to 4 weeks (Delayed). With smoked tobacco, induction (1A2) starts in 3 days and reverses in about 1 week.

INHIBITORS
InHibition increases substrate levels (High), happening within Hours (Hurried). Inhibition reverses as soon as the inhibitor is cleared from the body (five half-lives of the inhibitor).

SUBSTRATES
"Victims" of inducers and inhibitors

1A2 inducers
- Ψ **Tobacco/Cannabis** (faster on/off)
- Ψ Carbamazepine
- Ψ Phenytoin

1A2 inhibitors
- Ψ **Fluvoxamine**
- Ciprofloxacin

1A2 substrates
- Ψ Asenapine
- Ψ **Clozapine**
- Ψ Duloxetine
- Ψ Olanzapine
- Ψ **Ramelteon**
- Ψ Thiothixene

2B6 inducers
- Ψ Carbamazepine
- Rifampin
- **HIV MEDS**

2B6 inhibitors
- Ψ Orphenadrine (Norflex)

2B6 substrates
- **HIV MEDS**
- **CANCER MEDS**
- Ψ Bupropion
- Ψ Ketamine
- Ψ Methadone
- Ψ Selegiline

2C9 inducers
- **Rifampin**
- Ψ St John's Wort

2C9 inhibitors
- **Fluconazole**

2C9 substrates
- Ψ Valproate (VPA)

2C19 inducers
- Ψ Phenobarbital
- Rifampin
- Apalutamide

Ultrarapid metabolizer (UM) genotype (10% of population)

2C19 inhibitors
- Ψ **Cannabidiol** (CBD)
- **Fluconazole**
- Ψ Fluoxetine
- Ψ Fluvoxamine

Poor metabolizer (PM) genotype (10% of population)

2C19 substrates
- Ψ Citalopram
- Ψ Diazepam
- Ψ Escitalopram
- Ψ Phenobarbital
- Ψ Phenytoin
- Ψ Sertraline
- Ψ Methadone
- Warfarin

2D6 inducers
None

Ultrarapid Metabolizer (UM) genotype (5% of population)

2D6 inhibitors
- Ψ **Bupropion**
- Ψ Duloxetine
- Ψ **Fluoxetine**
- Ψ **Paroxetine**
- Quinidine

Poor metabolizer (PM) genotype (10% of population)

2D6 substrates
- Ψ **Tricyclics (TCAs)**
- Ψ Aripiprazole
- Ψ Atomoxetine
- Ψ Brexpiprazole
- Ψ Bupropion-OH
- Ψ Codeine *PRODRUG*
- Ψ Deutetrabenazine
- Ψ Dextromethorphan
- Ψ Duloxetine
- Ψ Haloperidol
- Ψ Iloperidone
- Ψ **Perphenazine**
- Ψ **Pimozide**
- Ψ Risperidone
- Tamoxifen *PRODRUG*
- Ψ Tetrabenazine
- Ψ **Thioridazine**
- Ψ Tramadol *PRODRUG*
- Ψ Vortioxetine

3A4 inducers
- Ψ **Carbamazepine**
- Ψ Modafinil
- Ψ **Phenobarbital**
- Ψ **Phenytoin**
- Rifampin
- Ψ St John's Wort

3A4 inhibitors
- **Protease Inhibitors (HIV)**
- Clarithromycin
- Diltiazem
- Grapefruit juice
- **Ketoconazole**
- **Itraconazole**
- Ψ **Nefazodone**
- Verapamil

3A4 substrates
- **Immunosuppressants**
- **Progestins**
- Ψ Alprazolam
- Ψ Aripiprazole
- Ψ Brexpiprazole
- Ψ Buprenorphine
- Ψ **Buspirone**
- Ψ Carbamazepine
- Ψ Cariprazine
- Ψ Chlordiazepoxide
- Ψ Clonazepam
- Ψ **Fentanyl**
- Ψ **Flibanserin**
- Ψ **Lemborexant**
- Ψ **Lumateperone**
- Ψ **Lurasidone**
- Ψ Pimavanserin
- Ψ Pimozide
- Ψ **Quetiapine**
- Sildenafil
- **Simvastatin**
- Ψ Suvorexant
- Tadalafil
- Ψ Valbenazine
- Ψ **Vilazodone**

UGT inducers
- Ψ Carbamazepine
- Estrogens
- Ψ Phenobarbital
- Ψ Phenytoin
- Rifampin

UGT inhibitors
- Ψ **Valproate (VPA)**

UGT substrates
- Ψ **Lamotrigine**
- Ψ **Lumateperone**

Lithium levels

Decreased by:
- Acetazolamide
- Ψ Caffeine
- Mannitol
- Theophylline
- Ψ Topiramate
- Ψ Zonisamide

Increased by:

Thiazides:
- HCTZ
- Chlorthalidone

NSAIDS:
- Celebrex
- Ibuprofen
- Indomethacin
- Naproxen
- Diclofenac

ACE Inhibitors "-prils"

ARBs "-sartans"

Antimicrobials:
- Tetracyclines
- Metronidazole

UGT and lithium visual mnemonics are explained in the *Visualize to Memorize* edition *Cafer's Mood Stabilizers & Antiepileptics*

Ψ = CNS meds (psychoactive)

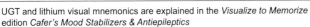

Pharmacokinetic Drug-Drug Interactions with included medications highlighted

INDUCERS

InDuction decreases (Down) substrates slowly, over 2 to 4 weeks* (Delayed).

Ψ Armodafinil	(3A4) weak
Apalutamide (prostate cancer)	2C19, 3A4 & (2C9)
Ψ Cannabis	1A2 fast
Chargrilled meat	1A2
Ψ Carbamazepine (Tegretol)	3A4, 2B6 & (1A2)
Efavirenz (HIV)	3A4, 2B6
Enzalutamide (prostate cancer)	3A4, 2C9 & 2C19
Estradiol	UGT
Ψ Modafinil	3A4
Nevirapine	2B6 (3A4)
Ψ Phenobarbital (Luminal)	3A4 (1A2), (2B6, 2C9) & UGT
Ψ Phenytoin (Dilantin)	3A4 (1A2), (2B6), UGT
Ψ Primidone (Mysoline) metab to phenobarb	3A4 (1A2), (2B6, 2C9) & UGT
Rifampin (Rifadin)	2C19, 3A4, 2B6, 2C9 (1A2) & UGT
Ritonavir (HIV)	2B6 (2C19) (1A2, 2C9)
Ψ St John's Wort	1A2, 2C9 & 3A4
Ψ Tobacco	1A2 fast
Ψ Topiramate ≥200 mg	(3A4)

inDuction reverses gradually over a few weeks* after the inducer is discontinued.

*With smoking (tobacco or cannabis), induction is faster (a few days).

Lithium levels

Decreased by:

Acetazolamide
Ψ Caffeine
Mannitol
Theophylline
Ψ Topiramate
Ψ Zonisamide (weak)

Increased by:

Benazepril
Celecoxib
Chlorthalidone
Diclofenac
Doxycycline
Enalapril

Etodolac
HCTZ
Ibuprofen
Indomethacin
Irbesartan Lisinopril
Tetracycline

Losartan
Metronidazole
Minocycline
Naproxen
Olmesartan
Ramipril
Valsartan

With high-dose aspirin, Depakote (VPA) will be stronger than suggested by total VPA level because aspirin (highly protein-bound) bumps VPA off of albumin.

INHIBITORS

InHibition increases substrate levels (High). Inhibition happens within Hours (Hurried).

Amiodarone	(2C9, 2D6, 3A4)
Ψ Asenapine	(2D6) weak
Ψ Bupropion	2D6
Ψ Cannabidiol	2C19, UGT (multi) weak
Cimetidine	1A2, (3A4)
Ciprofloxacin	1A2, (3A4)
Clarithromycin	3A4
Clopidogrel	(2B6)
Darunavir (HIV)	3A4, (2D6)
Diltiazem	3A4, (2D6)
Ψ Duloxetine	2D6
Efavirenz (HIV)	2C9, 2C19
Erythromycin	3A4
Esomeprazole	(2C19) weak
Ψ Fluoxetine	2D6, 2C19
Ψ Fluvoxamine (Luvox)	1A2, 2C19, & (3A4, 2C9)
Grapefruit juice	3A4
Isoniazid	(3A4) weak
Indinavir	3A4
Itraconazole	3A4
Ketoconazole	3A4, (2C19)
Ψ Methadone	(2D6) weak
Ψ Modafinil	(2C19) weak
Nelfinavir	3A4
Omeprazole	2C19
Ψ Nefazodone	3A4
Ψ Orphenadrine	2B6
Ψ Paroxetine	2D6
Quinidine	2D6, (3A4)
Ritonavir	3A4 Black Box
Ψ Sertraline ≥150mg	(2D6)
Terbinafine	2D6
Ψ Thioridazine	2D6
Ψ Valproate (VPA)	UGT-1A & -2B
Voriconazole	3A4,2C19,(2C9)
Verapamil	3A4, (1A2)

InHibition is reversed as soon as the inhibitor is cleared, which will be about 5 half-lives after it is discontinued.

UGT & UGT-1A refer to UGT1A4.
UGT-2B refers to UGT2B15.

( ) = weak inducer/inhibitor; less susceptible substrate

Ψ = CNS medication (psychoactive)

SUBSTRATES

"Victims" of inducers and inhibitors

In general, substrates that are metabolized through only one pathway are more vulnerable to drug interactions. For drugs metabolized by multiple CYPs, strong inDuction of a single CYP is likely to reduce substrate levels, but inHibition of one CYP is unlikely to significantly increase substrate levels.

Apixaban	3A4
Atazanavir (HIV)	3A4
Ψ Alprazolam	3A4
Ψ Amitriptyline	2D6, 2C19
Amlodipine	3A4
Ψ Amoxapine	2D6
Ψ Amphetamine salts	(2D6)
Ψ Aripiprazole	2D6, 3A4
Ψ Armodafinil	3A4
Ψ Asenapine	(1A2)
Ψ Atomoxetine	2D6, (2C19)
Atorvastatin	3A4
Avanafil	3A4
Ψ Brexpiprazole	2D6, 3A4
Ψ Buprenorphine	3A4
Ψ Bupropion	2B6; 2D6 (OH-)
Ψ Buspirone	3A4, (2D6)
Ψ Caffeine	1A2 (etc)
Ψ Carbamazepine	3A4
Ψ Cariprazine	3A4, (2D6)
Ψ Carisoprodol	2C19
Carvedilol	2D6 (etc)
Celecoxib	2C9, (3A4)
Ψ Chlordiazepoxide	3A4
Ψ Chlorpromazine	2D6, (1A2, 3A4)
Ψ Citalopram	2C19, (3A4,2D6)
Clarithromycin	3A4
Ψ Clomipramine	2D6, 2C19, 1A2
Ψ Clonazepam	3A4
Clopidogrel	2C19, (3A4)
Ψ Clozapine	1A2 (2D6, etc)
Ψ Codeine *2D6 prodrug	*2D6, (3A4)
Ψ Cyclobenzaprine	1A2, (2D6, 3A4)
Cyclophosphamide	2B6, 2C19
Cyclosporine	3A4 (etc)
Ψ Desipramine	2D6, (1A2)
Ψ Deutetrabenazine	2D6
Ψ Dextromethorphan	2D6 (etc)
Ψ Diazepam	2C19, 3A4
Diclofenac	multi
Diltiazem	3A4 (2C19,3A4)
Ψ Doxepin	2D6, 2C19 (etc)
Ψ Donepezil	(2D6, 3A4)
Ψ Duloxetine	2D6, 1A2
Efavirenz (HIV)	2B6, 3A4
Ψ Escitalopram	2C19, (3A4,2D6)
Esomeprazole	2C19, (3A4)
Estradiol	1A2, 2C9, 3A4
Ψ Eszopiclone	3A4
Ψ Fentanyl 3A4 Black Box	3A4 (etc)
Flecainide	2D6, 1A2
Ψ Flibanserin 3A4 Black Box	3A4, 2C9, 2C19
Ψ Fluoxetine	2D6, 2C9 (etc)
Ψ Fluphenazine	2D6
Ψ Flurazepam	3A4
Fluvastatin	2C9 (2B6, 3A4)
Ψ Fluvoxamine	2D6, 1A2
Ψ Galantamine	(2D6, 3A4)
Glimepiride	2C9
Glipizide	2C9
Glyburide	2C9
Ψ Guanfacine	3A4
Ψ Haloperidol	2D6, 3A4, (1A2)
Ψ Hydrocodone Black Box	3A4
Ifosfamide	2B6 (& others)
Ψ Iloperidone	2D6, (3A4)
Ψ Imipramine	2D6, 2C19 (etc)
Ψ Ketamine	2B6, 2C9, 3A4
Ψ Lamotrigine	UGT
Lansoprazole	2C19, 3A4
Ψ Lemborexant	3A4
Ψ Levomilnacipran	3A4, (2D6)
Ψ Lorazepam	UGT-2B (VPA)

Losartan	2C9, 3A4
Ψ Loxapine	(1A2, 2D6,3A4)
Ψ Lumateperone	3A4, UGT-1A
Ψ Lurasidone *contraind*	3A4
Medroxyprogesterone	3A4
Meloxicam	2C9, (3A4)
Ψ Meperidine Black Box	3A4
Ψ Methadone	3A4, 2B6, (etc)
Ψ Methamphetamine	2D6
Metoprolol	2D6, (2C19)
Mexiletine	1A2, 2D6
Ψ Midazolam	3A4, (2B6)
Ψ Mirtazapine	2D6, 3A4, 1A2
Ψ Modafinil	3A4 (2D6)
Nevirapine	3A4 (2B6, 2D6)
Ψ Nefazodone	3A4; 2D6 mCPP
Nifedipine	3A4, (2D6)
Norethindrone	3A4
Ψ Nortriptyline	2D6 (etc)
Ψ Olanzapine	1A2; (2D6)
Omeprazole	2C19 (etc)
Ψ Oxazepam	UGT-2B (VPA)
Ψ Oxycodone	3A4, (2D6)
Pantoprazole	2C19,(2D6, 3A4)
Ψ Paroxetine	2D6
Ψ Perphenazine	2D6 (etc)
Ψ Phenobarbital	2C19,(2C9)
Ψ Phenytoin	2C9, 2C19,(3A4)
Ψ Pimavanserin	3A4
Ψ Pimozide	2D6, 3A4 (1A2)
Piroxicam	2C9
Ψ Promethazine	(2B6, 2D6)
Propafenone	2D6, (1A2, 3A4)
Ψ Propofol	2B6 (etc)
Ψ Propranolol	2D6, 1A2,(2C19)
Ψ Protriptyline	2D6
Ψ Quetiapine	3A4, (2D6)
Ψ Ramelteon	1A2 (3A4,2C19)
Ψ Risperidone	2D6, (3A4)
Rivaroxaban	3A4
Ψ Selegiline	2B6 (etc)
Ψ Sertraline	2C19 (2B6,2D6)
Sildenafil	3A4, (etc)
Simvastatin	3A4
Ψ Suvorexant	3A4
Tacrolimus	3A4
Tadalafil	3A4
Tamoxifen *2D6 prodrug	*2D6, 3A4, 2C9
Ψ Tasimelteon	1A2, 3A4
Ψ Temazepam	UGT-2B (VPA)
Ψ Tetrabenazine	2D6
Theophylline	1A2, (3A4)
Ψ Thioridazine	2D6, (2C19)
Ψ Thiothixene	1A2
Ψ Tiagabine	3A4
Ψ Tizanidine	1A2
Tolbutamide	2C9, (2C19)
Ψ Tramadol *2D6 prodrug*	3A4,(2D6*; 2B6)
Ψ Trazodone	3A4 (2D6 mCPP)
Ψ Triazolam	3A4
Ψ Trifluoperazine	1A2
Ψ Trimipramine	2D6, 2C19, 3A4
Ψ Valproate (VPA)	(multi); Aspirin*
Ψ Valbenazine	3A4 (2D6)
Vardenafil	3A4
Ψ Venlafaxine	2D6, 3A4,(2C19)
Ψ Vilazodone	3A4,(2C19,2D6)
Vincristine	3A4
Voriconazole	2C9, 2C19, 3A4
Ψ Vortioxetine	2D6, 3A4, etc
Warfarin	2C9, 2C19,(3A4)
Ψ Zaleplon	(3A4)
Ψ Zolpidem	3A4 (etc)

Cafer's Psychopharmacology | cafermed.com

Neurotransmitters

Here is a simplified overview of neurotransmitters in the brain that are relevant to antidepressants. Serotonin, norepinephrine, dopamine, and histamine are referred to as <u>monoamine neurotransmitters</u> because they contain a single amine group ($-NH_2$). The monoamine neurotransmitters serotonin and dopamine are implicated in most psychiatric disorders.

For an in-depth explanation of how neurotransmitters influence mood and how drugs affect neurotransmitters. I recommend *Stahl's Essential Psychopharmacology:Neuroscientific Basis and Practical Applications.* Dr. Stahl's book is a classic—great for visual learners. *Prescriber's Guide: Stahl's Essential Psychopharmacology* is also required reading.

Neurotransmitter	Abbrev	Normal activity	Low activity	High activity	Comments
Serotonin (5-hydroxytryptamine)	5-HT	"Serenity" Calmness Satisfaction Euthymic mood Normal sleep	Depression Anxiety OCD	Sexual dysfunction, muscle twitching, hyperreflexia, dilated pupils, restlessness, gastrointestinal distress/nausea, serotonin syndrome, hallucinations (LSD)	Most antidepressants are serotonergic, i.e., enhance 5-HT neurotransmission.
Norepinephrine	NE	Energy, motivation, ability to focus and respond to stress	Fatigue Inattention Sexual dysfunction Hypotension	Insomnia, anxiety, nausea, loss of appetite, hypertension, seizure, dilated pupils	NE is also known as noradrenaline. Stimulants increase noradrenergic (NE) activity. Some antidepressants are noradrenergic.
Dopamine	DA	Motivation, ability to experience pleasure and strong emotions	Anhedonia, inattention, sexual dysfunction, parkinsonism, akathisia, dystonia, neuroleptic malignant syndrome (NMS), restless legs syndrome, antiemetic	Mania, euphoria, agitation, anger, aggression, chemical "high", paranoia, auditory hallucinations, compulsive behaviors, hypersexuality, insomnia, nausea, dilated pupils	Think pleasure, passion, paranoia. Drugs of abuse, colloquially known as "dope", cause euphoria by spiking DA in the nucleus accumbens. Many stimulants and Parkinson's disease medications are dopaminergic.Only a few antidepressants are dopaminergic.
Acetylcholine	ACh	"Rest and digest" parasympathetic activity, normal cognitive function	"Dry as a bone" - Constipation, urinary retention, dry mouth; "Mad as a hatter" - confusion, delirium with visual hallucinations; dilated pupils, tachycardia	"SLUDGE" - salivation, lacrimation, urination, diaphoresis, GI upset (including diarrhea), emesis; constricted pupils	Acetylcholine acts on muscarinic and nicotinic receptors. What are commonly described as "anticholinergic" effects would be more accurately termed "antimuscarinic".
Histamine	H	Alertness	Sedation Weight gain	Allergic reaction, pruritus, excessive gastric acid secretion	H_1 antihistamines are used for sleep and allergies; H_2 antihistamines (ranitidine, etc) reduce stomach acid; The H_3 antihistamine pitolisant (Wakix) promotes wakefulness.

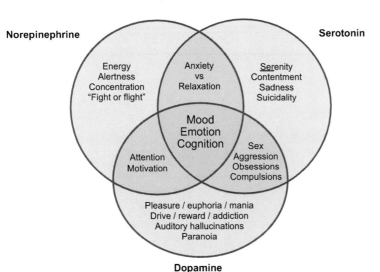

Selective serotonin reuptake inhibitors (SSRIs) block 5-HT transporters without significantly blocking DA or NE transporters. Serotonin-norepinephrine reuptake inhibitors (SNRIs) block 5-HT and NE transporters. The monoamine oxidase inhibitors (MAOIs) block the breakdown of all monoamine neurotransmitters, which is why MAOIs are more powerful antidepressants.

Serotonin & Dopamine

"Technically, the only two things you enjoy"

Most tricyclic antidepressants (TCAs) contribute anticholinergic (antimuscarinic) and antihistaminergic side effects.

Class	Abbrev	Antidepressant	$/mo	Comments
Tricyclic Antidepressant	TCA	Amitriptyline (ELAVIL) —┐ metabolized Nortriptyline (PAMELOR) ◄─┘ to Imipramine (TOFRANIL) ─┐ Desipramine (NORPRAMIN) ◄─┘ Clomipramine (ANAFRANIL) for OCD Doxepin 10 mg (generic) for sleep Doxepin 3 mg, 6 mg (SILENOR) for sleep Protriptyline (VIVACTIL) Maprotiline (LUDIOMIL) Amoxapine (ASENDIN) Trimipramine (SURMONTIL)	$10 $10 $10 $20 $200 $10 $400 $75 $50 $25 $100	TCAs are older antidepressants, rarely used for depression today. They are prescribed at low dose for insomnia and migraine prevention. TCAs are famous for anticholinergic side effects (constipation, dry mouth, urinary retention, confusion), orthostatic hypertension, weight gain, sedation, and sexual dysfunction. Not good for the elderly. Fatal in overdose due to disruption of cardiac conduction. There are significant differences between members of the TCA class—some are sedating, while others are energizing. Weight gain may be large.
Selective Serotonin Reuptake Inhibitor	SSRI	Sertraline (ZOLOFT) Escitalopram (LEXAPRO) Citalopram (CELEXA) Fluoxetine (PROZAC) Paroxetine (PAXIL) Fluvoxamine (LUVOX) for OCD	$5 $5 $5 $5 $5 $25	SSRIs are considered first-line treatment for depression and anxiety disorders. Side effects include sexual dysfunction, GI distress (nausea, diarrhea), headache, and fatigue. Possibility of modest weight gain with long term use. Risk of hyponatremia and impaired platelet functioning
Serotonin (5-HT) & Norepinephrine (NE) Reuptake Inhibitor	SNRI	Duloxetine (CYMBALTA) Venlafaxine ER (EFFEXOR XR) ─┐ Desvenlafaxine (PRISTIQ) ◄─┘ Levomilnacipran (FETZIMA) Milnacipran (SAVELLA) for fibromyalgia	$20 $10 $40 $350 $350	SNRIs are better for pain than are SSRIs. SNRIs may cause a dose-dependent increase in blood pressure due to noradrenergic (NE) activity. Compared to SSRIs, SNRIs are less likely to cause weight gain with long-term.
Norepinephrine Reuptake Inhibitor	NRI	Atomoxetine (STRATTERA) for ADHD	$300	For ADHD; Not considered an antidepressant. Rare risk of serious hepatic injury
"Atypical Antidepressants" Norepinephrine & Dopamine (DA) Reuptake Inhibitor	NDRI	Bupropion (WELLBUTRIN) TID Bupropion SR (WELLBUTRIN SR) Bupropion XL (WELLBUTRIN XL) Solriamfetol (SUNOSI) for somnolence	$30 $20 $20 $700	Stimulating. Modest weight loss and decreased urge to smoke. Improved sexual functioning. Risk of seizures at high dose.
Noradrenergic & Specific Serotonergic Antidepressant	NaSSA	Mirtazapine (REMERON)	$10	Great for sleep and stimulation of appetite. At higher dose, noradrenergic (NE) activity is more prominent (stimulating). Weight gain is common, but less prominent than with amitriptyline.
Serotonin Antagonist & Reuptake Inhibitor	SARI	Trazodone (DESYREL) Nefazodone (SERZONE)	$5 $75	Trazodone is widely prescribed at low dose as a sleep medication. Nefazodone, rarely prescribed, is less sedating.
Serotonin Modulator & Stimulator	SMS	Vilazodone (VIIBRYD) Vortioxetine (TRINTELLIX)	$200 $300	Less likely to cause weight gain or sexual dysfunction than SSRIs. Both off-patent in 2022
Monoamine Oxidase Inhibitor (non-selective)	MAOI	Phenelzine (NARDIL) Tranylcypromine (PARNATE) Isocarboxazid (MARPLAN)	$50 $250 $750	Potentially fatal if combined with tyramine rich foods (hypertensive crisis) or other serotonergic medications (serotonin syndrome). Effective for treatment-resistant depression
Selective MAO-B Inhibitor (transdermal)	MAOI patch	Selegiline transdermal (EMSAM) for depression	$1600	OK to combine with tyramine-rich foods with the lowest dose (6 mg) patch.
NMDA Receptor Antagonist		Ketamine (KETALAR) - intravenous Esketamine (SPRAVATO) - nasal	$10 $5000	Schedule III controlled anesthetic, rapidly effective for treatment-resistant depression
Neurosteroid		Brexanolone (ZULRESSO)	$34000	Approved for postpartum depression. Given as an IV infusion over 60 hours. Excessive sedation is possible.
Medical food		L-Methylfolate (DEPLIN)	$200	Active form of folate, add-on to an antidepressant
Herbal	SJW	St John's Wort	$25	For mild depression only. Inducer of several CYP enzymes

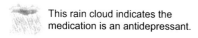 This rain cloud indicates the medication is an antidepressant.

 The asterisk means the medication is considered (or can be properly referred to as) an antidepressant, but is not typically prescribed for depression. Examples include clomipramine for OCD, fluvoxamine (Luvox) for OCD, trazodone (Desyrel) for insomnia, and milnacipran (Savella) for fibromyalgia.

Not an antidepressant   Some medications have mechanisms resembling depression medication but are not properly referred to as "antidepressants". Examples include the NRI atomoxetine (Strattera) and the NDRI solriamfetol (Sunosi).

With an antidepressant, improvement of mood can occur within the first two weeks, but it will take 4 to 6 weeks to achieve maximal benefit. About 60% of individuals experiencing a major depressive episode will respond to their first antidepressant. If no benefit is seen by 2 weeks, stay the course (if no side effects) because there is no advantage in switching to another antidepressant (Bschor et al, 2018). There is no disadvantage to switching antidepressants at 2 weeks either, so if the patient insists, go for it. Following resolution of a single depressive episode, the antidepressant should generally be continued for a year to consolidate recovery. For recurrent depressive episodes, long-term maintenance treatment may be indicated.

For adults, reasonable **first-line antidepressants** include:

First-line antidepressant	Class	Choose when	Sexual dysfunction	~ Cost/ month	Comments
Escitalopram (LEXAPRO)	SSRI	Depression with anxious distress	Yes	$5	Start 10 mg once daily (AM or PM). Usual maintenance dose is 10 to 20 mg. FDA max is 20 mg, but can go up to 60 mg for OCD (Stahl 2016). Always superior to citalopram (Celexa).
Sertraline (ZOLOFT)	SSRI	Depression with anxious distress	Yes	$5	Start 50 mg once daily (AM or PM). FDA max is 200 mg, but can go up to 400 mg for OCD (Stahl, 2016). More likely to cause nausea and diarrhea than Lexapro.
Bupropion (WELLBUTRIN)	NDRI	Depression with fatigue and oversleeping; comorbid ADHD or tobacco use disorder	No	$20	For XL formulation, start 150 mg AM; Max is 450 mg. For SR formulation, start 100 mg BID; Max 200 mg BID. The IR formulation (TID) is not recommended due to risk of seizure.
Mirtazapine (REMERON)	NaSSA	Depression with insomnia and loss of appetite	No	$10	Start 15 mg HS. FDA max is 45 mg, although 60 mg is safe. Higher doses are *less* sedating.

For first-episode depression, it is customary to start with an SSRI. For adults, no SSRI is clearly more effective than others, although escitalopram (Lexapro) has a slight advantage over the others for tolerability, and possibly for efficacy. For children, fluoxetine (Prozac) has the best evidence. For adults, escitalopram and sertraline (Zoloft) are preferred because they have fewer drug-drug interactions compared to fluoxetine or paroxetine (Paxil). Although quite safe, citalopram (Celexa) is a bit riskier than the other SSRIs due to mild QT prolongation, for which FDA lowered the recommended maximum from 60 mg to 40 mg. There is no reason to choose citalopram over escitalopram.

If the patient is not eating or sleeping, consider starting with mirtazapine (Remeron). If insomnia is prominent but weight gain is not desired, consider choosing an SSRI plus trazodone (Desyrel) 50 mg at bedtime, PRN or scheduled ($4). The FDA max for trazodone is 400 mg, but prescribed doses rarely exceed 200 mg.

For depressed patients with fibromyalgia or other types of chronic pain, an SNRI like venlafaxine (Effexor) or duloxetine (Cymbalta) would be a reasonable first-line choice. Effexor XR is dosed 75–225 mg QD. Cymbalta is 30–60 mg QD (FDA max 120 mg).

Treatment-resistant depression (TRD) is defined as failure of two 6-week antidepressant trials. For TRD, trying a third antidepressant is no more effective than placebo. Augmenting the antidepressant is twice as effective as placebo (Zhou et al, 2015). Lithium (0.5–0.8 mmol/L) and aripiprazole (Abilify) 5–15 mg are the top choices for augmentation. Other proven options include quetiapine (Seroquel) 100–300 mg HS, risperidone (Risperdal) 0.5–3 mg HS and liothyronine (Cytomel, T3 thyroid hormone) 50 mcg. There is moderate evidence for adding olanzapine (Zyprexa) 5–15 mg or buspirone (Buspar) 5–15 mg BID–TID. About 50% of TRD cases are actually bipolar disorder (Francesca et al, 2014), for which lithium or lamotrigine (Lamictal) are superior to antidepressants in preventing the next depressive episode.

Intravenous ketamine or intranasal esketamine are quickly effective for TRD. Electroconvulsive therapy (ECT) has the highest rate of response and remission of any form of antidepressant treatment.

All antidepressants have a <mark>black box warning</mark> of increased suicidal thoughts and behavior in children, adolescents and young adults. Increased risk of completed suicide has not been established. For adults beyond age 24, incidence of suicidal thoughts does not exceed placebo. For those age 65 and older, antidepressants decrease suicidal thoughts. In reduction of suicide risk, lithium is superior to antidepressants.

For children and adolescents, antidepressants (SSRIs, SNRIs) show more prominent benefit for anxiety than for depression (Locher et al, 2017).

All antidepressants have the potential to induce a "switch" to mania, usually in the context of undiagnosed bipolar disorder. Patients with known bipolar disorder suffering a depressive episode may be treated with an antidepressant combined with a mood stabilizer or an antipsychotic. Upon successful treatment of a bipolar depressive episode, consider tapering off the antidepressant after a few months to avoid destabilization of mood over the long term.

Following a Mediterranean diet can improve acute depression and prevent future depressive episodes (Jacka et al 2017; Parletta et al, 2017). 30–60 minutes of light therapy every morning can produce benefits comparable to medication for seasonal and non-seasonal depression (Penders et al, 2016). All depressed patients should be screened for hypothyroidism—ordering a serum TSH level is sufficient.

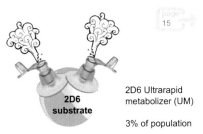

Almost all antidepressants are metabolized, at least in part, by CYP2D6. For patients with a 2D6 ultrarapid metabolizer (UM) genotype (3%), non-response to a wide range of antidepressants (at standard doses) is possible.

2D6 substrate

2D6 Ultrarapid metabolizer (UM)

3% of population

page 15

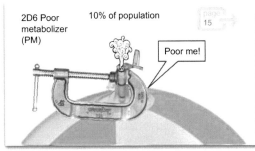

2D6 Poor metabolizer (PM)

10% of population

page 15

Poor me!

For the 10% of individuals who are 2D6 poor metabolizers (PM), antidepressant levels may be higher than expected, possibly leading to side effects. For a known 2D6 PM, it is recommended to dose the following at half-strength: tricyclics (TCAs), vortioxetine (Trintellix), and atomoxetine (Strattera).

The antidepressants not metabolized by 2D6:
► Desvenlafaxine (Pristiq)
► Selegiline (EMSAM patch)

Other antidepressants unlikely to be significantly affected by 2D6 interactions include citalopram (Celexa), escitalopram (Lexapro), sertraline (Zoloft), levomilnacipran (Fetzima), and vilazodone (Viibryd).

Serotonergic medications commonly decrease sexual desire, disrupt the sexual pleasure response, and increase latency to orgasm. Here are some drugs ranked (approximately) from worst to best in regard to sexual dysfunction:

- ❖ Paroxetine (Paxil) - the worst, > 70% of patients
- ❖ Sertraline (Zoloft) > 60% - *"so soft"*
- ❖ Escitalopram (Lexapro) and citalopram (Celexa) ~ 60%
- ❖ Fluoxetine (Prozac) ~ 60%
- ❖ Venlafaxine (Effexor) ~ 60%
- ❖ Fluvoxamine (Luvox) - least among the SSRIs but still > 50%
- ❖ Duloxetine (Cymbalta) - least among the SNRIs
- ❖ Vortioxetine (Trintellix) - minimal at 10 mg (44% at > 10 mg)
- ❖ Vilazodone (Viibryd) - slightly more than placebo
- ❖ Placebo - up to 30% sexual dysfunction
- ❖ Trazodone - possible enhancement (and risk of priapism)
- ❖ Nortriptyline and Desipramine (TCAs without serotonergic effects)
- ❖ Nefazodone (Serzone) - possible enhancement
- ❖ Mirtazapine (Remeron) - possible enhancement
- ❖ Bupropion (Wellbutrin) - enhances sexual functioning (female > male)
- ❖ Buspirone (BuSpar) - enhances sexual functioning (female > male)

About half of individuals taking <u>antipsychotics</u> also experience sexual dysfunction, particularly with antipsychotics that elevate prolactin like haloperidol (Haldol), risperidone (Risperdal), and paliperidone (Invega). Among antipsychotics, aripiprazole (Abilify) is the least likely to cause sexual dysfunction, followed by ziprasidone (Geodon), and quetiapine (Seroquel). <u>Mood stabilizers</u> are generally unlikely to cause sexual dysfunction. Lamotrigine (Lamictal) does not have sexual side effects.

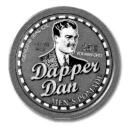

Dapoxetine is a short acting SSRI available in over 50 countries (but not the US) for PRN treatment of premature ejaculation. Paxil could be used PRN for this purpose, off-label. Also, the OTC cough suppressant dextromethorphan (DXM) can be used to delay orgasms via serotonergic mechanism.

Anticholinergic Burden Scale (Risk of CNS impairment/dementia) – "mad as a hatter"

Anticholinergic load should be minimized with older adults. Dose should be taken into consideration when estimating risk.

	3 Points (worst)	2 points	1 point (mild)	0 points
TCA Antidepressants	Amitriptyline, Clomipramine, Doxepin ≥ 50 mg, Imipramine, Maprotiline, Protriptyline, Trimipramine	Desipramine (Norpramin) Doxepin ≤ 25 mg (Sinequan) Nortriptyline (Pamelor)	Amoxapine (Asendin) Doxepin ≤ 10 mg (Sinequan)	Doxepin ≤ 6 mg (Silenor)
Other Antidepressants	N/A	Paroxetine (Paxil) - *"Paxil packs it in"* (constipation as a peripheral anticholinergic effect)	Citalopram (Celexa) Fluoxetine (Prozac) MAOIs Mirtazapine (Remeron)	SNRIs, Other SSRIs, Bupropion (Wellbutrin), Trazodone, Nefazodone, Vilazodone (Viibryd), Vortioxetine (Trintellix)
Antipsychotics (and other D2 blockers)	<u>Low potency FGAs:</u> Chlorpromazine (Thorazine) Promethazine (Phenergan) Thioridazine (Mellaril)	<u>Intermediate potency FGAs:</u> Loxapine (Loxitane) Molindone (Moban) Perphenazine (Trilafon) <u>SGAs:</u> Clozapine (Clozaril) Olanzapine (Zyprexa)	<u>High potency FGAs:</u> Fluphenazine (Prolixin) Haloperidol (Haldol) Pimozide (Orap) Prochlorperazine (Compazine) Thiothixene (Navane) Trifluoperazine (Stelazine) <u>SGAs:</u> Pimavanserin (Nuplazid) Quetiapine (Seroquel)	<u>SGAs:</u> Aripiprazole (Abilify) Asenapine (Saphris) Brexpiprazole (Rexulti) Cariprazine (Vraylar) Iloperidone (Fanapt) Lurasidone (Latuda) Paliperidone (Invega) Risperidone (Risperdal) Ziprasidone (Geodon)
Antihistamines	Cyproheptadine (Periactin) Diphenhydramine (Benadryl) Doxylamine (Unisom) Meclizine (Antivert) Hydroxyzine (Vistaril)	Chlorpheniramine (Chlor-Trimeton),	Cetirizine (Zyrtec) Cimetidine (Tagamet) Fexofenadine (Allegra) Loratadine (Claritin) Ranitidine (Zantac)	Levocetirizine (Xyzal)
Anticholinergics for OAB	Oxybutynin (Ditropan)	Tolterodine (Detrol)	Fesoterodine (Toviaz) Solifenacin (Vesicare)	Darifenacin (Enablex) Trospium (Sanctura)
Other Anticholinergics	<u>Atropine</u> (injected) Benztropine (Cogentin) Dicyclomine (Bentyl) Hyoscyamine (Levsin) Scopolamine (Transderm Scōp) Trihexyphenidyl (Artane)	Amantadine (Symmetrel) <u>Atropine</u> eye drops	Ip<u>ratropium</u> inhaler (<u>Atrovent</u>) Note that ip<u>ratropium</u> is like an inhaled form of <u>atropine</u> (the strongest anticholinergic)	Glycopyrrolate (Robinul)* *Strong anticholinergic but does not cross blood-brain barrier; Therefore it causes constipation but not cognitive problems.
Muscle relaxants	Carisoprodol (Soma) Orphenadrine (Norflex)	Cyclobenzaprine (Flexeril) Baclofen (Lioresal)	Methocarbamol (Robaxin)	Metaxalone (Skelaxin) Tizanidine (Zanaflex)
Sedatives	See antihistamines	See antihistamines	Diazepam (Valium) Temazepam (Restoril)	**Other benzodiazepines Z-drugs; barbiturates; melatonin
Mood stabilizers; Antiepileptics	N/A	Carbamazepine (Tegretol)	Lithium Oxcarbazepine (Trileptal)	Other anticonvulsants
Other	N/A	Cimetidine (Tagamet) Codeine Metoclopramide (Reglan) Pseudoephedrine (Sudafed)	Buspirone (Buspar) Pramipexole (Mirapex)	Antihypertensives, cognitive enhancers and ADHD stimulants; atomoxetine, ondansetron, tramadol, ropinirole

Compiled from many sources. There are at least 10 published anticholinergic risk/burden scales (including Beers criteria) which differ substantially in the estimation of anticholinergic load for certain medications.

**These sedatives may impair cognition, but not by anticholinergic effect.

Serotonin syndrome, better understood as serotonin toxicity, is a rare condition that can occur when serotonergic drugs are combined, especially with monoamine oxidase inhibitors (MAOIs). The mechanism involves serotonin overload in the brain stem. 50% of cases onset within 2 hours of adding the offending serotonergic. Only 25% of cases persist longer than 24 hours. 70% of cases resolve within 24 hours.

15% of SSRI overdoses lead to serotonin toxicity. Overdoses of a combination of a SSRI plus a MAOI have a 50% likelihood of causing serotonin syndrome.

Although it may rarely progress to multi-organ failure and death, serotonin syndrome is not as dangerous as the Neuroleptic Malignant Syndrome (NMS) caused by antipsychotic medications. Refer to pages 26–27 for a head-to-head comparison of 5-HT toxicity and NMS.

The diagnosis of 5-HT Syndrome is defined by the Hunter Serotonin Toxicity Criteria with 84% sensitivity and 97% specificity. The criteria focus on clonus, ocular clonus, and hyperreflexia.

On physical exam, the sufferer of 5-HT toxicity may appear uncomfortable and twitchy. Deep tendon reflexes may be very brisk. Try to elicit clonus by flexing the patient's foot and watching for rhythmic contractions of the ankle. Assess for ataxia through observation of gait, Romberg testing, and point-to-point testing.

Be careful if combining antidepressants with other medications that have serotonergic properties:

- ❖ dextromethorphan (DXM) – cough suppressant
- ❖ tramadol (Ultram) – pain medication (SNRI + weak opioid)
- ❖ methadone – opioid
- ❖ fentanyl – opioid
- ❖ meperidine (Demerol) – opioid
- ❖ metaxalone (Skelaxin) – muscle relaxant, MAOI activity
- ❖ cyclobenzaprine (Flexeril) – tricyclic muscle relaxant (unlikely)
- ❖ St. John's wort – herbal antidepressant
- ❖ LSD ("acid") – hallucinogen
- ❖ MDMA (ecstasy) – a common cause of serotonin toxicity
- ❖ linezolid (Zyvox) – an antimicrobial with MAOI activity
- ❖ methylene blue (Urelle) – urinary tract antiseptic

Mascots of ❖ red medications are featured in Chapter 7 - Serotonergics.

Despite an FDA warning, the risk of serotonin syndrome with a triptan migraine medication (Imitrex, Maxalt, etc) is miniscule, if not nonexistent. Orlova et al (2018) estimated the risk at about 1 in 10,000 person-years of exposure to a triptan plus an SSRI/SNRI. Serotonin syndrome is hypothesized to involve 5-HT$_{2A}$ and 5-HT$_{1A}$ receptors, while triptans are agonists at 5-HT$_{1B}$ and 5-HT$_{1D}$ receptors.

Combining SSRIs, combining SNRIs, or combining an SSRI with an SNRI makes no sense therapeutically, but is unlikely to cause serotonin toxicity at standard doses. Switching between SSRIs and SNRIs can generally be done without a washout period. Since fluoxetine (Prozac) has a long half-life, consider waiting a few days after stopping it before starting the replacement serotonergic antidepressant.

Treatment of 5-HT toxicity involves stopping the offending agent and aggressive cooling of high fever. In some cases, medications with anti-serotonergic activity may be helpful, such as the antihistamine cyproheptadine (Periactin) or the antipsychotic chlorpromazine (Thorazine).

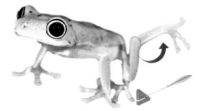

"Twitchy frog"

Hyperreflexia

Antidepressant Combinations

Reasonable combos (although not necessarily effective):

- ► Antidepressant + lithium
- ► Antidepressant (excluding nefazodone) + quetiapine (Seroquel)
- ► Escitalopram or sertraline + aripiprazole (Abilify) or risperidone (Risperdal)
- ► SSRI + buspirone (Buspar)
- ► Trazodone + other antidepressant (excluding nefazodone)
- ► Trazodone + doxepin for sleep
- ► Fluoxetine + olanzapine (Zyprexa)
- ► SSRI + bupropion (Wellbutrin)
- ► Nortriptyline + escitalopram or sertraline
- ► SNRI + mirtazapine (Remeron) - "California Rocket Fuel" (page 55)
- ► MAOI + TCA without serotonergic activity— nortriptyline, desipramine, maprotiline, trimipramine = "Non-Disparaged MAOI Tagalongs"

"Bad" combinations

- ► 2 SSRIs
- ► 2 SNRIs
- ► SSRI + SNRI
- ► 2 TCAs
- ► SNRI + TCA
- ► Fluoxetine or paroxetine (strong 2D6 inhibitors) with 2D6 substrates (including all TCAs)
- ► Bupropion + noradrenergic TCA or SNRI
- ► Antidepressant + St John's wort
- ► SSRI or SNRI + tramadol (Ultram)
- ► Mirtazapine + clonidine or guanfacine
- ► Atomoxetine + SNRI, bupropion, fluoxetine or paroxetine

Dangerous combinations

- ► MAOI + other antidepressants, excluding those without serotonergic effects (trazodone, bupropion, nortriptyline, desipramine, maprotiline, trimipramine)

History lesson: A high-profile case of serotonin syndrome occurred in 1984. Libby Zion, an 18-year-old college freshman taking the MAOI phenelzine presented to the ER and was treated with meperidine (Demerol) to control "strange jerking movements" (think twitchy frog). She was hospitalized, developed a fever of 107°F, and died of a heart attack within hours.

Her father, an attorney, believed her death was the result of overworked resident physicians. In 1989 New York state adopted the "Libby Zion Law" which limited medical residents to 80 hours per week. In 2003 all accredited medical training institutions adopted a similar regulation, limiting residents to 80 hours per week and 24 consecutive hours.

Serotonin (5-HT) Syndrome and Neuroleptic Malignant Syndrome are rare psychiatric emergencies. These syndromes should be considered when an individual taking several psychotropic medications becomes acutely ill. Since some symptoms overlap, here is a head-to-head comparison.

NMS - "can't Bend(er)"

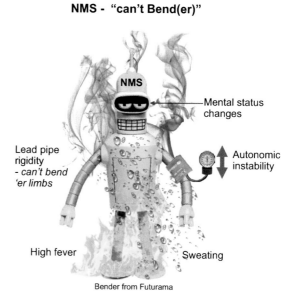

Mental status changes

Lead pipe rigidity - *can't bend 'er limbs*

Autonomic instability

High fever

Sweating

Bender from Futurama

5-HT "twitchy frog" syndrome

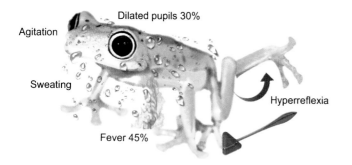

Dilated pupils 30%

Agitation

Sweating

Hyperreflexia

Fever 45%

	Serotonin Syndrome		Neuroleptic Malignant Syndrome (NMS)
Mechanism	Serotonin (5-HT) overload in the brain stem		Dopamine blockade in the hypothalamus (fever) and nigrostriatal pathway (rigidity)
Usual onset	Within 24 hours of combining antidepressants (or other serotonergics)		Within 30 days of starting or increasing an antipsychotic (anti-dopaminergic) or stopping a dopaminergic drug
Cardinal features	Myoclonic jerks > 50% Hyperreflexia > 50% Mental status changes > 50% Shivering > 50%		High fever 100% by definition Rigidity 100% by definition Mental status changes 99% Elevated or labile BP most
Fever	45%		Yes; Temp > 40°C (104°F) in 40% of cases
Autonomic instability	35% tachycardia 35% HTN 15% hypotension		99% overall 88% tachycardia 70% labile BP
Mental status change	51% confusion 50% restlessness/hyperactivity/agitation 29% unresponsiveness (may evolve to coma)		Confusion is the first symptom to present in 82% of cases, and may evolve to mutism, profound encephalopathy and coma.
Muscle rigidity	51% and less severe than with NMS		100% by definition; "lead pipe rigidity"
Motor activity	Hyperkinesia (restlessness/hyperactivity)		Bradykinesia (slowness of movement)
Hyperreflexia	52%		No
Clonus	23% - Examine for repetitive dorsiflexion of the ankle in response to one forcible dorsiflexion. Go to *cafermed.com/clonus* to see how its done.		No
Tremor	43%	You could *clone us* (clonus)	Less prominent
Ataxia	40%		Uncommon
Shivering	> 50%		Uncommon
...with chattering teeth or bruxism	15%		No
Sweating (diaphoresis)	Common		Common
Sialorrhea (hypersalivation)	Often prominent		< 15%
Eyes	30% dilated pupils; 20% unreactive pupils; Ocular clonus is possible as seen on *cafermed.com/clonus*.		Usually not affected; Go to *cafermed.com/crisis* to see oculogyric crisis, a manifestation of dystonia which may co-occur with NMS.

continued...

	Serotonin Syndrome	Neuroleptic Malignant Syndrome (NMS)
Nature of syndrome	Can be referred to as serotonin toxicity because it is a true toxidrome, caused by excess serotonin in a concentration-dependent way; Some cases are mild.	An idiosyncratic reaction, not a toxidrome; All cases of NMS are serious. Partial, early, or aborted presentations of NMS cases were described as forme fruste, especially with low potency antipsychotics. Rigidity may be absent or milder with clozapine.
Typical evolution	Rapid onset; May have prodrome of nausea and diarrhea; Serotonin toxicity may be mild to severe.	First: Mental status changes (confusion, mutism, catatonia); Second: Rigidity; Third: Fever and BP lability; Peak severity in as little as 3 days
Mortality	1% mortality if treated; When fatal, it is usually due to extreme fever, leading to the same complications as seen with NMS.	Fatal if untreated; 10% mortality when treated; Renal failure from rhabdomyolysis, heart attack, respiratory failure (from chest wall rigidity), DVT/pulmonary embolism, dehydration, electrolyte imbalance, disseminated intravascular coagulation (DIC), liver failure, seizures
Resolution	70% of cases completely resolve within 24 hours.	If not fatal, NMS typically resolves slowly over 1 to 2 weeks.
Most likely culprits	15% of SSRI overdoses lead to 5-HT toxicity; 50% incidence when overdosing on combo SSRI + MAOI; Clomipramine, imipramine are most likely among TCAs.	High potency 1st gen antipsychotics (FGAs); Haldol is responsible for 44% of cases. Long-acting injectable FGAs—haloperidol decanoate (Haldol D) and fluphenazine decanoate (Prolixin D)—pose an even higher risk.
Non-antidepressant/ antipsychotic culprits	LSD ("Acid") / MDMA (Ecstasy) / Dextromethorphan (DXM) / L-Tryptophan / Metaxalone (Skelaxin) / Linezolid (Zyvox) / Methylene blue (Urelle) · St. John's Wort / Tramadol (Ultram) / Meperidine (Demerol) / Fentanyl (Duragesic) / Methadone (Dolophine) / Buspirone (Buspar) - unlikely / Triptans (Imitrex, Maxalt, etc) - highly unlikely	Antiemetics that are D2 blockers: - Metoclopramide (Reglan) - Prochlorperazine (Compazine) - Promethazine (Phenergan) - Trimethobenzamide (Tigan) / TCA that blocks D2 receptors: - Amoxapine (Asendin) · Dopamine depleting agents - Reserpine (Serpasil) - Tetrabenazine (Xenazine) - Deutetrabenazine (Austedo) - Valbenazine (Ingrezza)
Lithium?	Lithium may contribute to 5-HT syndrome, although unlikely	Lithium may contribute to NMS.
Caused by stopping...	N/A	Stopping a dopaminergic antiparkinson medication (e.g., levodopa) can induce NMS. This variety of NMS is referred to as parkinsonism-hyperpyrexia syndrome or "withdrawal-emergent hyperpyrexia and confusion".
Relatively low risk medications	Rarely caused by a lone antidepressant. Not caused by buspirone or triptans. Highly unlikely to be caused by mirtazapine, trazodone, cyclobenzaprine or lithium.	Low potency 1st gen antipsychotics—chlorpromazine (Thorazine) and thioridazine (Mellaril); 2nd gen antipsychotics—clozapine (Clozaril), quetiapine (Seroquel), olanzapine (Zyprexa)
Leukocytosis	Less prominent	> 75% of cases have WBC > 12,000
Creatinine kinase (CK) elevation	Less prominent	90% show creatine kinase (CK) over 3x upper limit of normal (ULN). CK of over 5x ULM is diagnostic of rhabdomyolysis (skeletal muscle breakdown), which can lead to renal failure and disseminated intravascular coagulation (DIC). The normal range of CK is 22 to 198 units/Liter. CK is also called creatine phosphokinase (CPK).
Management	Discontinue the contributing medication(s). Aim to normalize vital signs.	ICU admission, rapid cooling and hydration. Stop the antipsychotic or restart the dopaminergic med.
Potentially helpful meds	Benzodiazepines for agitation / Cyproheptadine (anti-serotonergic antihistamine) / Methysergide (anti-serotonergic migraine medication)	Bromocriptine (DA agonist) / Amantadine (DA agonist, NMDA antagonist) / Dantrolene (direct acting muscle relaxant)
Risk factors	Combinations of serotonergics, use of street drugs	Iron deficiency, dehydration, catatonia, Lewy body dementia, genetically reduced function of D2 receptors, rapid dose escalation, males under age 40
Incidence	Severe 5-HT toxicity is rare. Mild toxicity is more common.	Quite rare - About 1 in 5,000 on antipsychotics
Sequelae	None, although delirium may persist for a few days	Memory problems (although usually temporary)
Differential diagnosis	Serotonin discontinuation syndrome (withdrawal) in the context of cross-tapering/titrating antidepressants. Anticholinergic toxicity, which manifests as dry, flushed skin ("dry as a bone, red as a beet") rather than diaphoresis.	Alcohol withdrawal, thyrotoxicosis, sepsis, heat stroke, tetanus, acute hydrocephalus, status epilepticus
Formal diagnosis	Google Hunter criteria, which focuses on clonus (spontaneous or inducible), ocular clonus, and hyperreflexia	Defined by DSM 5; Severe rigidity and high fever are both necessary to make the diagnosis.
Notes	Some experts prefer the term serotonin toxicity to more accurately reflect the condition as a dose-dependent form of 5-HT poisoning.	Neuroleptic, a synonym of antipsychotic, refers to something that "grabs ahold of nerves". Idiopathic NMS (with no identifiable culprit drug) is called malignant catatonia.

Thanks to Ahmed Eid Elaghoury MD for contributing to this content.

QT prolongation
"Cutie heart"

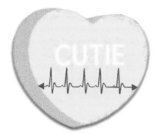

In this book, an ECG tracing like the one on this candy heart means that the medication prolongs QT interval.

On electrocardiogram (ECG), the QT interval, measured from the beginning of the QRS complex to the end of the T-wave, reflects the rate of electrical conduction through the ventricles as they contract and relax. The useful number for our purposes is the QT**c** interval, which is QT **c**orrected for heart rate, which takes into account that QT interval is naturally longer at slower heart rate.

ECG of Normal Sinus Rhythm

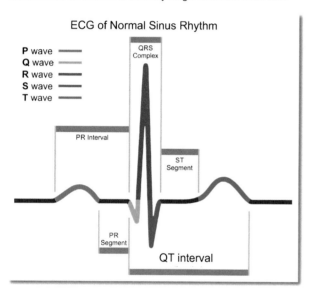

P wave
Q wave
R wave
S wave
T wave

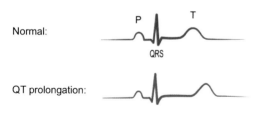

Normal:

QT prolongation:

QT prolongation is a delay in cardiac conduction that can trigger **Torsades de pointes** (French "twisting of points"). This may precede sudden death.

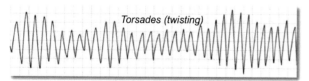

Torsades (twisting)

Many psychotropic medications prolong QT interval, including most antidepressants and antipsychotics. In overdose scenarios involving antidepressants or antipsychotics, QT interval is usually long, necessitating a trip to the ICU. As you will see in the next chapter, tricyclic antidepressants (TCAs) are particularly deadly in overdose due to disruption of cardiac conduction manifested by, among other measures, prolonged QT.

Roughly speaking, QTc > 460 milliseconds is long and QTc > 500 msec can be dangerous. An increase in QTc > 60 msec caused by a medication would be of concern.

The risk of torsades is the highest within the first few days of initiating treatment with a QT prolonger. For most drugs that prolong QT, the risk of torsades is so low that routine ECG screening is unnecessary. Although combining QT prolonging medications does prolong QT interval, the magnitude of the effect is likely to be tiny, with a very low probability of clinical consequences (Carlat Report, March 2018). However, it is prudent to check an ECG for patients taking high doses of multiple QT prolonging medications, or individuals with these risk factors:

Risk factors for QT prolongation
▶ Hypokalemia (low K+)
▶ Hypomagnesemia (low Mg+)
▶ Bradycardia
▶ Left ventricular hypertrophy

Patients with congenital long QT syndrome should not be given QT prolonging medications. Do not add a QT prolonging medication when QTc is near 500 msec.

QT prolongation by psychotropic medications:

Risk	Medication	Class
Highest	Thioridazine (Mellaril)	Antipsychotic
High	Pimozide (Orap)	Antipsychotic
	Ziprasidone (Geodon)	Antipsychotic
Moderate	Iloperidone (Fanapt)	Antipsychotic
	Chlorpromazine (Thorazine)	Antipsychotic
	Haloperidol (Haldol)*	Antipsychotic
	Amitriptyline (Elavil)	TCA
	Desipramine (Norpramin)	TCA
	Imipramine (Tofranil)	TCA
	Maprotiline (Ludiomil)	TCA
	Citalopram (Celexa)	SSRI
	Methadone (Dolophine)	Opioid
	Pitolisant (Wakix)	H3 antihistamine
Low risk except in combination or overdose	Most antidepressants Most antipsychotics	

*Intravenous haloperidol poses high risk of QT prolongation.

Due to the extent of QT prolongation caused by thioridazine (Mellaril), most psychiatrists avoid prescribing it. For healthy patients taking ziprasidone (Geodon), the author checks an ECG before exceeding the FDA maximum dose of ziprasidone (80 mg BID) or when combining 3 or more medications known to prolong QT interval. Check an ECG if a patient taking QT prolonging medications experiences palpitations or syncope/presyncope.

Other medications that prolong QT interval:

Class	Medication
Antiarrhythmic	Amiodarone (Cordarone)
	Flecainide (Tambocor)
	Quinidine (Cardioquin)
	Sotalol (Betapace)
Antimicrobial	Azithromycin (Zithromax)
	Ciprofloxacin (Cipro)
	Clarithromycin (Biaxin)
	Erythromycin (Erythrocin)
	Fluconazole (Diflucan)
	Hydroxychloroquine (Plaquenil)
	Levofloxacin (Levaquin)
Other	Cocaine
	Opioids (most) - generally mild except methadone
	Ondansetron (Zofran) - antiemetic (IV route)
	Propofol (Diprivan) - anesthetic

Tricyclic Antidepressants (TCAs)
[tri SIC lic] including the -triptylines [-trip ta LEEN]
"Tricycles tripped a line"

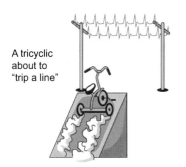

A tricyclic about to "trip a line"

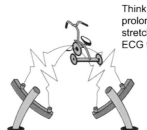

Think of QT prolongation as a stretching out of the ECG tracing.

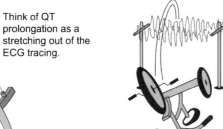

If QT interval is too long, Torsades de pointes may result.

The TCAs are older antidepressants, derived from the three-ringed chemical (imipramine) shown above. They work by inhibiting reuptake of serotonin (5-HT) and/or norepinephrine (NE). TCAs differ from newer SSRIs and SNRIs in that TCAs are "dirty drugs", non-selectively affecting several other neurotransmitter systems. Most TCAs are antihistaminic (sedation and weight gain) and anticholinergic (dry mouth, constipation, urinary retention, and confusion). They also block alpha-1 adrenergic (NE) receptors, which may lead to orthostatic hypotension.

Mechanistically, the prototypical TCA is like a combination of venlafaxine (SNRI), diphenhydramine (antihistamine and anticholinergic) and prazosin (alpha-1 blocker). This does not apply to all TCAs, which are a diverse bunch. Amitriptyline and imipramine are prototypical TCAs.

TCAs were largely replaced by SSRIs, which are cleaner (selective), without the antihistaminic and anticholinergic baggage. Unlike the diverse TCAs, SSRIs are pretty much homogenous, with similar efficacy and side effects. The main difference between members of the SSRI class are half-life and potential for kinetic interactions.

This chapter highlights the differences between members of the TCA class. Some TCAs are anxiety-reducing (amitriptyline, doxepin), while others can be energizing (nortriptyline, desipramine).

Clomipramine is highly serotonergic, whereas four TCAs have so little serotonergic activity that they could be safely coadministered with an MAOI— nortriptyline, desipramine, maprotiline, trimipramine = "Non-Disparaged MAOI Tagalongs".

TCAs are deadly in overdose, some more dangerous than others. Overdose on a ten-day supply of a TCA can be life-threatening owing to disturbance of cardiac conduction. This is seen on EKG as prolongation of the QT interval and other forms of conduction delay. The exception is clomipramine, which is relatively benign in overdose.

Compared to SSRIs, TCAs are less likely to contribute to serotonin syndrome, with clomipramine as an exception.

Although TCAs are not addictive or abusable, they are reported on the basic urine drug screen (UDS). False positive tricyclic screens can be caused by carbamazepine (Tegretol), oxcarbazepine (Trileptal), cyclobenzaprine (Flexeril), quetiapine (Seroquel), chlorpromazine (Thorazine), thioridazine (Mellaril), and at toxic doses, diphenhydramine (Benadryl).

The muscle relaxant cyclobenzaprine (Flexeril) is a tricyclic by structure. Single-drug overdose on cyclobenzaprine is less dangerous than overdose on a prototypical TCA.

Rx	TCA	Cost	Sed	Wt	ACh	NE	5-HT	Comments
#1	Amitriptyline (ELAVIL) _metabolized to_	$10	+++	+++	+++	++	+++	Calming (as opposed to drive-enhancing). The most weight gain among TCAs. Highly anticholinergic so not good for the elderly.
#2	Nortriptyline (PAMELOR)	$10	+	+	+	++++	-	Drive-enhancing. The least orthostatic hypotension of TCAs. Active metabolite of amitriptyline.
#3	Doxepin (SILENOR)	$10 ($450)	+++	++	+++	++	+++	Highly antihistaminic. Effective for sleep at very low dose. 3 mg and 6 mg tablets are expensive. 10 mg capsules are cheap.
#4	Imipramine (TOFRANIL)	$15	++	++	++	++	+++	1st antidepressant approved in US. Metabolized to desipramine.
#5	Clomipramine (ANAFRANIL)	$380	+++	++	+++	-	++++	Highly serotonergic, for OCD only. The safest TCA in overdose.
#6	Desipramine (NORPRAMIN)	$15	+/-	+/-	+	++++	-	Energizing with minimal side effects. Exceptionally fatal in overdose. The only TCA likely to cause hypertension.
#7	Protriptyline (VIVACTIL)	$81	-	+/-	+++	++++	+/-	Energizing / drive-enhancing
#8	Maprotiline (LUDIOMIL)	$68	++	++	+	++++	-	Tetracyclic structure. Risk of inducing seizures.
#9	Amoxapine (ASENDIN)	$25	+	++	+/-	+++	++	Tetracyclic. Weak antipsychotic with potential to cause EPS.
#10	Trimipramine (SURMONTIL)	$88	+++	++	++	-	-	Highly sedating. Not a significant 5-HT or NE reuptake inhibitor. Antihistamine and 5-HT$_{2A}$ antagonist.

Rx – sales rank; Cost – month's supply (see GoodRx.com); Sed – sedation; Wt – weight gain;
ACh – anticholinergic; NE – noradrenergic (norepinephrine); 5-HT – serotonergic

Amitriptyline (ELAVIL)
am i TRIP ta leen / EL a vil

"Am I trippin' (off the) Elevator?"

❖ Tricyclic Antidepressant (TCA)
❖ Serotonin and norepinephrine reuptake inhibitor (SNRI)
❖ 5-HT₂ receptor antagonist
❖ 5-HT > NE

10 mg
<u>25</u>
50
75
100
150

FDA-approved for:
❖ Depression

Used off-label for:
❖ Neuropathic pain
❖ Migraine prevention
❖ Fibromyalgia
❖ Postherpetic neuralgia
❖ Insomnia

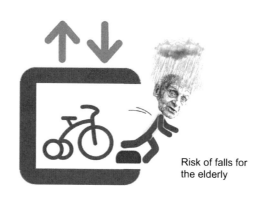

Risk of falls for the elderly

"*Elavil elevates your mood*". Introduced in 1961, amitriptyline (Elavil) was heavily prescribed prior to the arrival of SSRIs. Amitriptyline remains the most prescribed TCA, and is the #88 most prescribed drug in the US. It appears to be more effective than newer antidepressants (Cipriani et al, 2018). Off-label uses include headache prevention, fibromyalgia, and insomnia.

Amitriptyline is <u>anxiety-reducing</u> (as opposed to drive-enhancing). Amitriptyline is <u>not recommended for the elderly</u> because it is more anticholinergic and antihistaminic than the average TCA. This can lead to falls. Of the tricyclics, it is the most likely to cause <u>weight gain</u>, averaging about 15 pounds over 6 months—"*Am I fat now?*"

Amitriptyline is <u>highly anticholinergic</u>. <u>Dry mouth</u> (an anticholinergic effect) occurs in almost everyone who takes 50 mg or more nightly.

Although amitriptyline is not the deadliest TCA, it is the most prescribed. As a result, <u>over 40% of all antidepressant fatalities</u> are caused by amitriptyline. It <u>should not be prescribed to patients with a history of</u> <u>overdosing</u> on pills. Of 33,219 single-drug exposures to amitriptyline reported to Poison Control, there were 145 deaths (Nelson & Spyker, 2017). This equates to a mortality risk of 1 in 229. Multi-drug overdoses including amitriptyline are much more dangerous.

Amitriptyline is metabolized to nortriptyline, which has fewer side effects and fewer interactions. So, why are more scripts written for amitriptyline than for nortriptyline? Possibly because the side effect of sedation is not a bug, it's a feature—amitriptyline is often intended to double as a sleep medication.

Dosing: For <u>depression</u> start 10 or 25 mg HS and titrate slowly due to sedative effects. The usual maintenance dose for depression is 50–150 mg HS. Maximum is 300 mg HS for depression and 150 mg for other uses. The target dose range for <u>migraine prophylaxis</u> is 10–100 mg HS. For <u>neuropathic pain</u>, consider dispensing a bottle of 10 mg tabs and instruct the patient to take 10 mg HS for one week and increase the dose by 10 mg weekly until pain is improved, up to 50 mg HS while they wait for their follow-up visit. Taper gradually to discontinue. Consider dispensing less than a 30-day supply if the patient is at risk of overdosing.

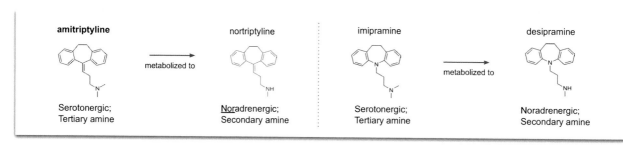

amitriptyline		nortriptyline	imipramine		desipramine
	metabolized to →			metabolized to →	
<u>S</u>erotonergic; Tertiary amine		<u>N</u>oradrenergic; Secondary amine	<u>S</u>erotonergic; Tertiary amine		<u>N</u>oradrenergic; Secondary amine

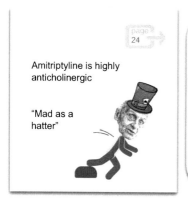

Amitriptyline is highly anticholinergic

"Mad as a hatter"

page 24 →

Dynamic interactions:
❖ Serotonergic
❖ Sedation/CNS depression
❖ Weight gain (worst of TCAs)
❖ QT prolongation (moderate)
❖ Anticholinergic (strong)
❖ Lowers seizure threshold (moderate)
❖ Hyponatremia
❖ Hypotension

Kinetic interactions:
❖ 2D6 substrate (major)
❖ 2C19 substrate

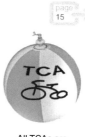

All TCAs are 2D6 substrates.

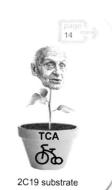

2C19 substrate

page 15 →

page 14 →

Nortriptyline (PAMELOR)
nor TRIP ta leen / PAM e lor

"North-tripping Pam"

❖ Tricyclic Antidepressant (TCA)
❖ Norepinephrine reuptake inhibitor (NRI)

10
25
50
75
mg

FDA-approved for:
❖ Depression

Used off-label for:
❖ Migraine prevention
❖ Smoking cessation
❖ ADHD
❖ Fibromyalgia
❖ Postherpetic neuralgia

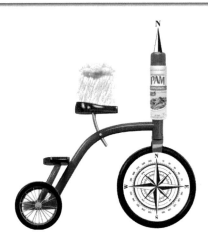

Nortriptyline (Pamelor) is the major active metabolite of amitriptyline. Sometimes nortriptyline is referred to as a second generation TCA (amitriptyline being the first generation). Nortriptyline is a norepinephrine reuptake inhibitor (NRI) with no significant serotonergic activity. It is similar to bupropion (Wellbutrin), although with more side effects and greater toxicity in overdose. Because it is not serotonergic, nortriptyline *could* be safely combined with an MAOI for refractory depression (Thomas & Shin et al, 2015).

Nortriptyline is arguably underutilized because it is superior to other TCAs in terms of safety and tolerability (Gillman, 2007). It has a relatively wide margin between therapeutic effects and side effects/toxicity. Nortriptyline causes the least orthostatic hypotension among the TCAs, so the individual is less likely to become lightheaded and fall—Pamelor *"keeps Pam's head pointed North"*. It can be effective for SSRI non-responders. It is one of two antidepressants (citalopram) with demonstrated benefit for post-stroke depression.

Not all TCAs combine well with SSRIs, but nortriptyline plus sertraline (Zoloft) or escitalopram (Lexapro) is considered a favorable pairing. Nortriptyline has been shown more effective than escitalopram for depression in individuals with high C-reactive protein, which is a general marker of inflammation (Uher et al, 2014).

Sedation from nortriptyline is by antihistamine effect. The label instructs to give nortriptyline at bedtime. Considering its stimulating properties, AM dosing may be more appropriate for some patients.

Nortriptyline has been used off-label for smoking cessation and ADHD, which is reasonable because its mechanism of action resembles that of atomoxetine (approved for ADHD) and bupropion (approved for smoking, used off-label for ADHD).

Think twice before prescribing nortriptyline to anyone at risk of overdosing on pills. Risk of mortality in single-drug overdose is only slightly less than with amitriptyline.

Initial milligram dose for nortriptyline is the same as amitriptyline and imipramine, although the FDA max for nortriptyline (150 mg) is lower than for amitriptyline/imipramine (300 mg).

Dosing: According to the label, the target dose for depression is 50–150 mg HS; Start: 25–50 mg HS and increase by 25–50 mg/day q 2–3 days; Max dose is 150 mg/day; May give in divided doses, or in AM; Use lower dose for elderly patients. Taper dose gradually to stop. Therapeutic serum range is about 50–150 ng/mL, which is easy to remember since the recommended dose range is 50–150 mg. Serum level does not necessarily correlate with clinical efficacy.

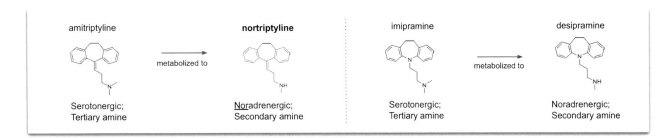

amitriptyline		nortriptyline		imipramine		desipramine
	metabolized to				metabolized to	
Serotonergic; Tertiary amine		Noradrenergic; Secondary amine		Serotonergic; Tertiary amine		Noradrenergic; Secondary amine

Therapeutic serum ranges are defined for desipramine, imipramine and nortriptyline —"mosquitos DINe on your blood".

Serum level does not necessarily correlate with clinical efficacy.

Dynamic interactions:
❖ QT prolongation (mild)
❖ Anticholinergic (moderate)
❖ Lowers seizure threshold (moderate)
❖ Sedation/CNS depression

Kinetic interactions:
❖ 2D6 substrate (major)
    - 2D6 ultra-rapid metabolizers may have undetectable serum levels of nortriptyline

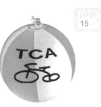

All TCAs are 2D6 substrates.

Doxepin (SILENOR)
DOX e pin / SIGH len or

"Box pins (for a) Silent night"

#239
1969
$10–$21 caps
$450–$550 tabs

❖ Tricyclic Antidepressant (TCA)
❖ NE & 5-HT reuptake inhibitor
❖ 5-HT$_2$ receptor antagonist
❖ Antihistamine (sedating)

10
25
50
75
100
150
Cheap

3
6
mg
Expensive

FDA-approved for:
❖ Depression (150–300 mg HS)
❖ Anxiety (150–300 mg HS)
❖ Insomnia (3–6 mg, branded Silenor)
❖ Pruritus (topical cream)

Used off-label for:
❖ Insomnia (10–25 mg generic Sinequan)

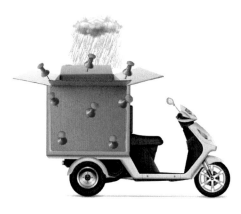

Doxepin (Sinequan) was released in 1969 as a tricyclic antidepressant (TCA). It is an incredibly strong antihistamine. It is available as a topical cream for pruritus.

Doxepin is rarely prescribed at antidepressant strength (150–300 mg capsules) but is commonly used at 10 mg for insomnia. The advantage of doxepin over other antihistamines for sleep is doxepin has minimal anticholinergic activity at a low dose. Traditional antihistamines such as diphenhydramine (Benadryl) and doxylamine (Unisom) are highly anticholinergic, as are the other sedating TCAs such as amitriptyline (Elavil) and clomipramine (Anafranil). In most circumstances, anticholinergic effects are undesirable. Anticholinergics constipate, cause xerostomia, impair cognition ("mad as a hatter") and increase risk of dementia with long-term use. Doxepin's advantage is lost at a high dose where it becomes highly anticholinergic.

Overdosing on a bottle of any full-strength TCA can be fatal, However, low dose Doxepin is safe to prescribe, even for patients at risk for suicidal overdose for whom you would never prescribe most TCAs. A 30-day supply of Doxepin 10 mg is only 300 mg, which would not kill a patient downing the full bottle (although 300 mg could theoretically be contributory to a fatal multidrug overdose).

The original trade name of the (now generic) doxepin capsule is Sinequan. A tiny dose doxepin tablet was released in 2017, branded as Silenor, available in 3 mg and 6 mg strengths. Generic 3 mg or 6 mg pills do not exist. Branded Sillenor costs about $15 per tablet, which is about $450 monthly. Compare this to 10 mg generic doxepin capsules, which are only $0.33 per capsule (about $10 monthly).

Generic doxepin (Sinequan) carries the same black box warning as all other antidepressants regarding suicidal thoughts and behaviors in children and young adults. Silenor (3 mg, 6 mg) does not have the boxed warning

Dosing: For depression or anxiety the target dose is 150–300 mg HS, starting at 25–75 mg HS; Max is 300 mg; May divide doses; Taper gradually to stop; For insomnia use 10 mg capsule HS; Max for insomnia is 50 mg, although if you stick with 10–20 mg then overdose on a 30-day supply will not be fatal; Avoid the 3 mg and 6 mg tabs (Silenor brand) due to cost.

$11–$21 caps

Doxepin (SINEQUAN)
DOX e pin / SIN e qwan

"Box pin Sine wave"

The original brand name of doxepin capsule was Sinequan, approved for depression and anxiety in the maintenance dose range of 150–300 mg HS.

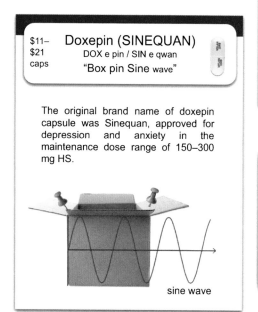

sine wave

Doxepin is a strong antihistamine

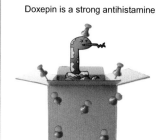

"Anti-HISSed-amine"

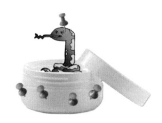

Doxepin 5% cream is approved as a topical antihistamine for pruritus, branded as Zonalon, priced at $300–$660 per tube. The cream may cause systemic symptoms including sedation and anticholinergic effects, especially if applied to > 10% of body surface. The cream is intended for no longer than 8 days of treatment.

Dynamic interactions:
❖ Serotonergic
❖ Sedation/CNS depression (strong)
❖ QT prolongation (mild)
❖ Anticholinergic (strong > 50 mg)
❖ Lowers seizure threshold (moderate)
❖ Hyponatremia
❖ Hypotension

Kinetic interactions:
❖ 2C19 substrate
❖ 2D6 substrate

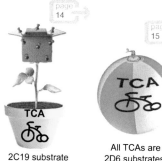

page 14
page 15

2C19 substrate

All TCAs are 2D6 substrates.

Cafer's Psychopharmacology | cafermed.com

1957	Imipramine (TOFRANIL)	❖ Tricyclic Antidepressant (TCA)	10
$21–$78	im IP ra meen / TOE fra nil	❖ 5-HT > NE reuptake inhibitor (SNRI)	25
	"I'm stopping it! (with) toffee"	❖ Antihistamine	50 mg

FDA-approved for:
❖ Depression
❖ Enuresis (bedwetting)

Used off-label for:
❖ Generalized anxiety disorder
❖ Panic disorder
❖ Chronic pain
❖ Sleepwalking
❖ Sleep terrors
❖ Confusional arousals

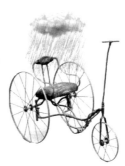

the oldest bicycle, representing he oldest antidepressant

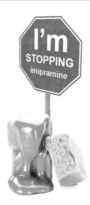

"I'm stopping it" due to side effects.

In 1957 imipramine (Tofranil) was released to the US market as the first antidepressant. It was widely prescribed prior to the arrival of better tolerated antidepressants. It is still prescribed for refractory depression.

Imipramine was originally synthesized in 1951 by tweaking the molecule of the antipsychotic chlorpromazine (Thorazine). At the time, these chemicals were classified as antihistamines. The antipsychotic effect of Thorazine was discovered in 1952. Imipramine was then tested as an antipsychotic but was ineffective for psychosis. Serendipitously, imipramine was found to relieve severe depression.

Imipramine is an example of a "dirty" chemical, i.e., it affects many neurotransmitter systems indiscriminately. It highly anticholinergic. Many patients report lightheadedness related to antagonism of alpha-1 adrenergic receptors, which causes orthostatic hypotension. Imipramine is a very poor choice for elderly patients who are at risk for falls.

Imipramine is considered a powerful antidepressant, more likely than others to lead to "switching" to mania when used for bipolar depression. Navarro et al (2019) found that 72% of nonresponders to venlafaxine (Effexor) showed remission of depression when changed to imipramine. By comparison, remission rate was only 39% when mirtazapine (Remeron)

was added to venlafaxine. In other words, imipramine was shown to outperform "California Rocket Fuel" (page 55).

Imipramine and clomipramine are the TCAs established as effective for panic disorder.

Imipramine was used to treat nocturnal enuresis because it shortens the duration of deep sleep, when bedwetting occurs. Other TCAs can be effective for enuresis, but imipramine is the only psychotropic medication FDA-approved for this indication. The other medication approved for enuresis is desmopressin (DDAVP), an antidiuretic derived from vasopressin.

The liver converts imipramine into desipramine (desmethyl-imipramine) as a metabolite. Desipramine (Norpramin) is a "cleaner" drug, affecting fewer neurotransmitter systems and causing fewer side effects. In terms of tolerability, *"desipramine is more desirable than imipramine"*.

Dosing: Dosing for imipramine is the same as for amitriptyline. For depression start at 10 or 25 mg HS and titrate slowly due to sedative effects. The usual maintenance dose for depression is 50–150 mg HS. Maximum is 300 mg HS (100 mg max for elderly patients); Taper gradually to stop. Therapeutic serum level is 150–300 ng/mL of combined imipramine plus desipramine.

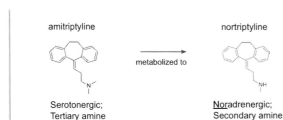

amitriptyline		nortriptyline	imipramine		desipramine
Serotonergic; Tertiary amine	metabolized to	Noradrenergic; Secondary amine	Serotonergic; Tertiary amine	metabolized to	Noradrenergic; Secondary amine

Therapeutic serum ranges are defined for desipramine, imipramine and nortriptyline —"mosquitos DINe on your blood".

Serum level does not necessarily correlate with clinical efficacy.

Dynamic interactions:
❖ Serotonergic (strong)
❖ Sedation/CNS depression (moderate)
❖ QT prolongation (mild)
❖ Anticholinergic (strong)
❖ Lowers seizure threshold (moderate)
❖ Hyponatremia (5-HT)
❖ Hypotension (strong)

Kinetic interactions:
❖ 2C19 substrate
❖ 2D6 substrate

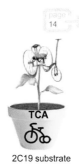

TCA

2C19 substrate

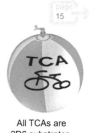

TCA

All TCAs are 2D6 substrates.

| 1990 $84–$239 | | Clomipramine (ANAFRANIL) kloe MIP ra meen / an AF ra nil "Anne Frank's Clompulsion" | ❖ Tricyclic Antidepressant (TCA) ❖ 5-HT > NE reuptake inhibitor (SNRI) ❖ Antihistamine | 25 50 75 mg |

FDA-approved for:
- ❖ Obsessive-compulsive disorder (OCD)

Used off-label for:
- ❖ Cataplexy (in narcolepsy)
- ❖ Confusional arousals
- ❖ Sleep terrors
- ❖ Sleepwalking

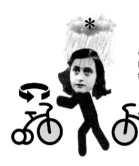

Obsessive-"Clompulsive" behavior of aligning tricycles

Clomipramine is one of four antidepressants (maprotiline, amoxapine, and bupropion IR) known to significantly <u>lower seizure threshold</u>, i.e., may predispose the individual to having a seizure. The risk is dose-dependent.

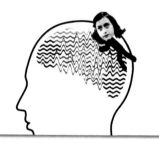

Clomipramine (Anafranil) was engineered from imipramine in the early 1960s. It was approved for treatment of depression in Europe in 1970, but not available in the US until 1990. This delay was because the FDA considered it just a "me too" drug of imipramine. Eventually, the FDA approved it for obsessive-compulsive disorder (OCD).

✱ Clomipramine is the only available TCA <u>not approved for depression</u>. It has been established as effective for <u>panic disorder</u>, off-label.

Clomipramine was considered the gold standard for treatment of OCD due to potent <u>serotonergic</u> activity. The other medication approved for OCD but not for depression is the SSRI fluvoxamine (Luvox), which is also highly serotonergic.

Due to side effects, clomipramine is considered a <u>third-line</u> OCD treatment after two trials of high-dose SSRIs have failed (Robert Hudak, MD). It may be somewhat more effective than SSRIs for OCD.

Clomipramine may be <u>the safest TCA</u>. Of 680 single-drug exposures to clomipramine reported to Poison Control, there were <u>no deaths</u> and only 44 major serious outcomes (Nelson & Spyker, 2017). Protriptyline (Vivactil) may be safer, but the sample size was small (77 exposures).

Dosing: For OCD start 25 mg QD, increase by 25 mg QD every 4–7 days for maximum of 200 mg in the first 2 weeks, then to FDA maximum maintenance dose of 250 mg. Give in divided doses with food during initial titration. Taper gradually to discontinue.

Dynamic interactions:
- ❖ Serotonergic (very strong)
- ❖ Sedation/CNS depression
- ❖ Weight gain (moderate)
- ❖ QT prolongation (mild)
- ❖ Anticholinergic (strong)
- ❖ Lowers seizure threshold (strong)
- ❖ Hyponatremia (5-HT)
- ❖ Antiplatelet effects (5-HT)

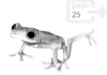

Clomipramine poses a particularly high risk of **serotonin toxicity** if combined with another serotonergic drug.

Kinetic interactions:

Multi-CYP
- ❖ 2C19 substrate
- ❖ 2D6 substrate
- ❖ 1A2 substrate
- ❖ 3A4 substrate

Multi-CYP substrates are less likely to be involved in clinically significant interactions.

page 25

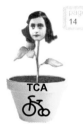

2C19 substrate

page 14
page 15

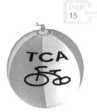

All TCAs are 2D6 substrates.

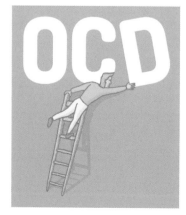

Serotonergic medications need to be dosed high to effectively treat obsessive-compulsive disorder. Citalopram (Celexa) is not a suitable SSRI for OCD due to QT prolongation at high dose.

Serotonergic medication	Class	FDA Maximum	Maximum for OCD (Stahl, 2016)
Clomipramine (Anafranil)	TCA	250 mg	250 mg
Fluvoxamine (Luvox)	SSRI	300 mg	450 mg
Escitalopram (Lexapro)*	SSRI	20 mg	60 mg
Fluoxetine (Prozac)	SSRI	80 mg	120 mg
Paroxetine (Paxil)	SSRI	60 mg	100 mg
Sertraline (Zoloft)	SSRI	200 mg	400 mg

*Off-label

Cafer's Psychopharmacology | cafermed.com

Desipramine (NORPRAMIN)

des IP ra meen / NOR pra min

"<u>Deceased</u> (No prayin', man)"

1963
$17– $50

❖ Tricyclic Antidepressant (TCA)
❖ <u>Nor</u>epinephrine reuptake inhibitor (NRI)

10
<u>25</u>
50
75
100
150
mg

FDA-approved for:
❖ Depression

Used off-label for:
❖ REM sleep behavior disorder
❖ ADHD

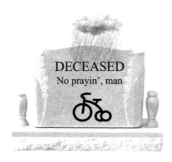

Released in 1963, desipramine (Norpramin) was once commonly prescribed, but is rarely used today. It is exceptionally <u>fatal in overdose</u>. Desipramine is an active metabolite of imipramine. In regard to side effects, *"desipramine is more <u>des</u>irable than imipramine"*.

Desipramine (and nortriptyline) have been referred to as <u>second generation TCA</u>s, making imipramine (and amitriptyline) first generations.

Desipramine is "<u>drive enhancing</u>" (stimulating), as opposed to "anxiety reducing". It can be described as a relatively selective <u>nor</u>epinephrinereuptake inhibitor (NRI). The trade name <u>Nor</u>pramin is fitting because it is the most potent <u>nor</u>adrenergic TCA. Don't confuse Norpramin with <u>nor</u>triptyline, which is also <u>nor</u>adrenergic.

Desipramine has the weakest antihistamine activity of all TCAs, making it <u>non-sedating</u>. While other TCAs are useful for treating insomnia, desipramine can cause insomnia. Recommended dosing is once daily in the <u>morning</u>. Unlike most other TCAs, desipramine causes <u>no weight gain, sexual dysfunction, or orthostatic hypotension</u>. It is the only TCA that can cause <u>hypertension</u>.

The observation that desipramine helped ADHD was the basis for development of the NRI atomoxetine (Strattera).

The main disadvantage of desipramine is risk of <u>mortality</u> in single-dose overdose, which appears to be <u>higher than any other antidepressant</u>. Out of 680 single-drug overdoses, there were 11 deaths, and 52 had major serious outcomes (Nelson & Spyker, 2017).

Therapeutic serum ranges are defined for <u>des</u>ipramine, <u>im</u>ipramine and <u>nor</u>triptyline—"mosquitos <u>DIN</u>e on your blood". On drug screens, desipramine can cause a false positive for amphetamine or LSD.

Dosing: Start 25–50 mg q AM and increase by 25–50 mg intervals every 2–3 days to target of 150–200 mg QD; Max is 300 mg; Taper gradually to stop. Therapeutic serum level is 150–300 ng/mL.

amitriptyline → nortriptyline

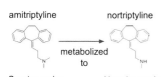

Serotonergic;
Tertiary amine

→ metabolized to →

<u>Nor</u>adrenergic;
Secondary amine

imipramine → **desipramine**

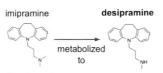

Serotonergic;
Tertiary amine

→ metabolized to →

Noradrenergic;
Secondary amine

Dynamic interactions:
❖ QT prolongation (moderate)
❖ Anticholinergic (moderate)
❖ Lowers seizure threshold (moderate)
❖ Hypertensive (unlike other TCAs)

Kinetic interactions:
❖ 2D6 substrate

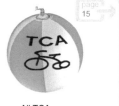

All TCAs are 2D6 substrates.

page 15

Protriptyline (VIVACTIL)

pro TRIP ta leen / viv ACT il

"Vivactil the ptero<u>dactyl</u>'s Pro tip (to lean)"

1966
$68–$181

❖ Tricyclic Antidepressant (TCA)
❖ <u>Nor</u>epinephrine reuptake inhibitor (NRI)

5
<u>10</u>
mg

FDA-approved for:
❖ Depression

Used off-label for:
❖ ADHD
❖ Narcolepsy (wakefulness promoter)
❖ Migraine prophylaxis
❖ Chronic pain
❖ Smoking cessation

As the trade name suggests, protriptyline (Vivactil) is a <u>stimulating</u> TCA. It is so energizing that it has been used to treat ADHD and to promote daytime wakefulness with narcolepsy. Protriptyline is safe to use with sleep apnea because it is a respiratory stimulant (the same can be said for fluoxetine, a relatively stimulating SSRI). Potential for weight gain is minimal. It appears to be <u>less toxic in overdose</u> than other TCAs, although sample size is small. Of 77 single-drug overdoses, there were no deaths and only 2 major serious outcomes.

Available since 1966, protriptyline is rarely prescribed, ranked #7 of 10 in TCA sales. Since 2000 it has been unavailable in several countries including the UK and Australia. Protriptyline is <u>the only TCA given in TID–QID</u> divided doses, but it could be dosed less frequently given its long half-life of about 80 hours.

I'm Viv<u>act</u>il the Pterodactyl. My <u>pro tip</u> is <u>to lean</u> like this.

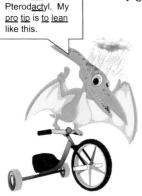

Dosing: Protriptyline has <u>uniquely low dosing among TCAs</u> due to its long half-life of about 80 hours. Protriptyline's dose range is 15 to 40 mg/day (divided TID–QID) compared to the usual TCA range of 25–300 mg/day. Therapeutic serum range for protriptyline is about 70–250 ng/mL is similar to other TCAs.

Dynamic interactions:
❖ QT prolongation (moderate)
❖ Anticholinergic (strong)
❖ Lowers seizure threshold (moderate)
❖ Hypotensive (moderate)

Kinetic interactions:
❖ 2D6 substrate

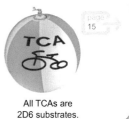

All TCAs are 2D6 substrates.

page 15

Amoxapine (ASENDIN)
a MOX a peen / a SEND in
"Ammo to Ascend"

❖ Tricyclic Antidepressant (TCA)
❖ Norepinephrine & Serotonin
Reuptake inhibitor
❖ NE > 5-HT
❖ D2 antagonist (weak)

25
50
100
150
mg

FDA-approved for:
❖ Depression

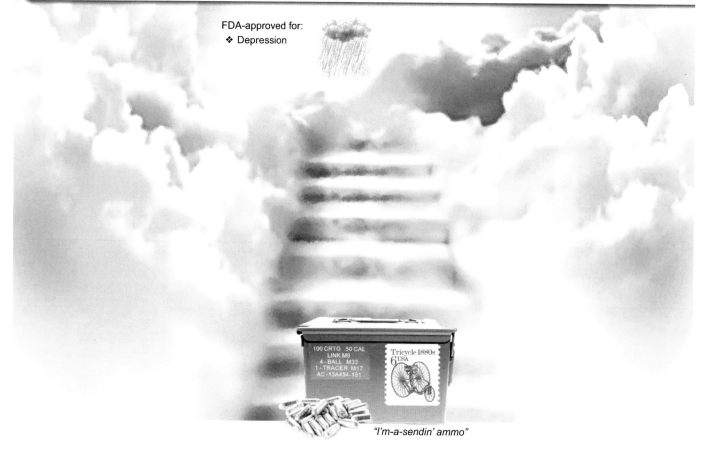

"I'm-a-sendin' ammo"

Although grouped with the tricyclic antidepressants (TCAs), amoxapine (Asendin) is actually a <u>tetracyclic antidepressant</u> (TeCA) by structure with four hydrocarbon rings. Amoxapine is rarely prescribed. It is <u>the least anticholinergic</u> of all TCAs.

Amoxapine is one of two antidepressants (trimipramine) that <u>block D2 dopamine receptors</u>. Dopamine antagonism gives amoxapine <u>weak antipsychotic</u> properties as well as risk of <u>extrapyramidal symptoms</u> (EPS) and prolactin elevation. The first generation antipsychotic (FGA) loxapine (Loxitane) is metabolized to amoxapine. Note that other drugs with the <u>-pine suffix</u> are antipsychotics (olanzapine, quetiapine, clozapine, asenapine, etc).

Out of 71 single-drug exposures reported to Poison Control, there 7 major serious outcomes including 1 death (Nelson & Spyker, 2017). This is a high mortality index, but due to small sample size it is undetermined whether amoxapine is actually more dangerous than the average TCA. Regardless, a bottle of amoxapine may provide the suicidal patient *"ammo to ascend"* to heaven.

Dosing: Target dose for depression is 200–300 mg HS or in divided doses; The label recommends starting at 50 mg BID–TID; Max is 400 mg/day if outpatient (600 mg/day if inpatient); Divide doses > 300 mg daily; Taper gradually to stop.

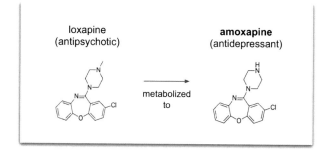

loxapine
(antipsychotic)

metabolized
to

amoxapine
(antidepressant)

Amoxapine has a high risk of inducing seizures.

Risk of seizures:
#1 Maprotiline (LUDIOMIL) highest risk
#2 **Amoxapine** (ASENDIN) high risk
#3 Clomipramine (ANAFRANIL) 1–3% risk
#4 Bupropion (WELLBUTRIN) IR 1–2% risk

In general, antidepressants (other than TCAs) have a slight <u>antiepileptic</u> effect at therapeutic dose.

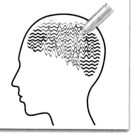

Dynamic interactions:
❖ Serotonergic
❖ Lowers seizure threshold (high risk)
❖ Extrapyramidal effects (D2 blocker)
❖ QT prolongation (mild)
❖ Anticholinergic (mild)
❖ Hypotensive (moderate)
❖ Hyponatremia (5-HT)

Kinetic interactions:
❖ 2D6 substrate

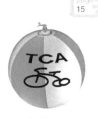

All TCAs are
2D6 substrates.

1976
$45–$84

Maprotiline (LUDIOMIL)
ma PRO ti leen / LU dee o mil
"Map telling Lude milf"

❖ Tricyclic Antidepressant (TCA)
❖ Norepinephrine reuptake inhibitor (NRI)

25
50
75
mg

FDA-approved for:
❖ Depression

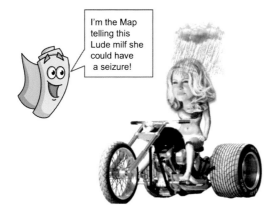

I'm the Map telling this Lude milf she could have a seizure!

Maprotiline (Ludiomil) is a tetracyclic antidepressant commonly classified as a TCA. It is a drive-enhancing norepinephrine reuptake inhibitor (NRI) without serotonergic effects.

Of all available antidepressants, maprotiline is the most likely to cause a seizure, although risk is less than 1 in 1,000 at standard dose assuming no other risk factors. Seizure risk can be minimized by slow titration. Since there is also a risk of bone marrow suppression, nortriptyline or desipramine is a better choice if you are looking for NRI tricyclic.

Dosing: Target dose for depression is 75–150 mg HS or in divided doses; Start 75 mg HS, may increase by 25 mg daily in 2-week intervals; Max is 150 mg for outpatient use (225 mg max for inpatient); Max for elderly is 75 mg; The label instructs a faster inpatient titration, though seizure risk will be higher; Taper gradually to stop.

Noradrenergic (NE) activity among TCAs:

Most:
Desipramine (NORPRAMIN)
Protriptyline (VIVACTIL)
Maprotiline (LUDIOMIL)

Least:
Clomipramine (ANAFRANIL)
Trimipramine (SURMONTIL)z

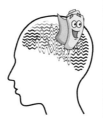

Antidepressants that lower seizure threshold:

#1 **Maprotiline** (LUDIOMIL) - highest risk of seizure
#2 Amoxapine (ASENDIN) - TCA
#3 Clomipramine (ANAFRANIL) - TCA
#4 Bupropion IR (immediate-release WELLBUTRIN)

Dynamic interactions:
❖ Lowers seizure threshold (worst among antidepressants)
❖ QT prolongation (moderate)
❖ Anticholinergic (moderate)

Kinetic interactions:
❖ 2D6 substrate

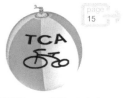

page 15

All TCAs are 2D6 substrates.

1979
$42 - $128

Trimipramine (SURMONTIL)
try MIP ra meen / SUR mon til
"Sermon 'til trimming"

❖ Tricyclic Antidepressant (TCA)
❖ 5-HT$_{2A}$ antagonist
❖ Antihistamine (sedating)
❖ D2 antagonist (antipsychotic)

25
50
100
mg

Sermon 'til trimming!

FDA-approved for:
❖ Depression

Trimipramine (Surmontil) is the least prescribed of the TCAs available in the US. You'll probably never see it in the wild.

Trimipramine's mechanism differs from other TCAs. It is not a significant 5-HT or NE reuptake inhibitor. It is mainly an antihistamine and 5-HT$_{2A}$ receptor antagonist. It is also one of two antidepressants (amoxapine) that block D2 dopamine receptors This gives it antipsychotic properties and the potential to cause extrapyramidal symptoms (EPS) and elevate prolactin. Trimipramine has a receptor binding profile similar to the antipsychotic clozapine (Clozaril).

Trimipramine can be highly sedating, which is an H$_1$ antihistaminic effect.

Dosing: Target dose for depression is 50–150 mg HS or in divided doses; Max is 200 mg/day for outpatients (300 mg/day for inpatients); Max for elderly patients is 100 mg; Taper gradually to stop.

Dynamic interactions:
❖ Sedation/CNS depression
❖ Extrapyramidal effects (D2 blocker)
❖ Hypotension
❖ Anticholinergic (strong)

Kinetic interactions:
❖ 2C19 substrate
❖ 2D6 substrate

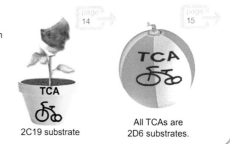

page 14 page 15

2C19 substrate

All TCAs are 2D6 substrates.

Toxicity of psychotropic medication in overdose

Listed from highest to lowest risk (approximate) of fatality in single-drug overdose:

Class		Medication	Mortality Index
TCA	Antidepressant	Desipramine (Norpramin) — *11 deaths from 680 overdoses*	141
TCA	Antidepressant	Amoxapine (Asendin)* — *1 death from 71 overdoses*	124
Combo		Perphenazine + amitriptyline (Triavil)	74
TCA	Antidepressant	Amitriptyline (Elavil), doxepin (Sinequan), imipramine (Tofranil)	~ 40
MAOI	Antidepressant	Phenelzine (Nardil), tranylcypromine (Parnate)	~ 35
Other		Aspirin	~35
TCA	Antidepressant	Nortriptyline (Pamelor)	~ 30
Other		Acetaminophen (Tylenol)	~25
Combo		Olanzapine + fluoxetine (Symbyax)	~25
SNRI	Antidepressant	Venlafaxine (Effexor)	9.7
AED	Mood stabilizer	Valproate (Depakote, Depakene)	8.1
NDRI	Antidepressant	Bupropion (Wellbutrin)	7.5
SGA	Antipsychotic	Olanzapine (Zyprexa), quetiapine (Seroquel), ziprasidone (Geodon)	~ 6–7
AED	Antiepileptic	Gabapentin (Neurontin)	5.8
AED	Mood stabilizer	Carbamazepine (Tegretol)	~ 5
SNRI	Antidepressant	Desvenlafaxine (Pristiq)	~ 5
OTC	Antihistamine	Diphenhydramine (Benadryl)	~ 5
SSRI	Antidepressant	Citalopram (Celexa), fluvoxamine (Luvox)	~ 4
Benzo	Anxiolytic	Benzodiazepines (alprazolam, clonazepam, lorazepam, etc)	3.4
NaSSA	Antidepressant	Mirtazapine (Remeron)	~ 3
SARI	Antidepressant	Nefazodone (Serzone)	~ 3
SGA	Antipsychotic	Risperidone (Risperdal)	2.5
AED	Mood stabilizer	Lamotrigine (Lamictal)	2.2
SNRI	Antidepressant	Duloxetine (Cymbalta)	2
SSRI	Antidepressant	Paroxetine (Paxil)	1.4
TCA	Antidepressant	Clomipramine (Anafranil), protriptyline (Vivactil)*	0–1
SNRI	Antidepressant	Levomilnacipran (Fetzima)*, milnacipran (Savella)	0–1
SARI	Antidepressant	Trazodone (Desyrel)	0–1
SMS	Antidepressant	Vilazodone (Viibryd), vortioxetine (Trintellix)*	0–1
SSRI	Antidepressant	Escitalopram (Lexapro), fluoxetine (Prozac), sertraline (Zoloft)	0–1
SGA	Antipsychotic	Aripiprazole (Abilify), lurasidone (Latuda)	0–1
AED	Antiepileptic	Oxcarbazepine (Trileptal), pregabalin (Lyrica)	0–1
SRA	Anxiolytic	Buspirone (Buspar) — *No deaths from 9,081 overdoses*	0–1

Mortality index = deaths per 10,000 single-drug exposures reported to Poison Control (about half of which were suicide attempts).

*Small sample size. Mortality index numbers are from Nelson & Spyker, 2017.

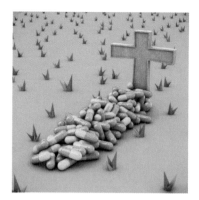

It is important for prescribers to have a general awareness of relative risk among medications and select drugs accordingly. <u>Multi-drug</u> overdoses are more serious. Certain drugs that are relatively benign in single-drug overdoses (e.g., benzodiazepines, quetiapine, gabapentin) are more dangerous when combined with or drugs or alcohol.

Patients presenting to the emergency department with a single-drug overdose on a drug with mortality index < 3 could probably be admitted directly to the behavioral health unit if there are no major mental status changes and ECG shows no cardiac conduction delay. Otherwise, most overdose patients should be admitted to the intensive care unit (ICU).

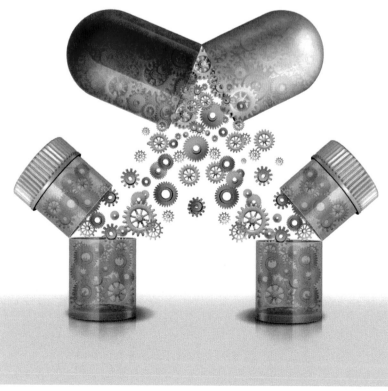

Cafermed.com discount code for
Cafer's Psychopharmacology:
Visualize to Memorize 270
Medication Mascots: **EMBIGGEN**

Selective Serotonin Reuptake Inhibitors (SSRIs)

SSRIs are the mainstay of treatment for depression, generalized anxiety disorder, panic disorder, and obsessive-compulsive disorder (OCD). By blocking serotonin transporters (SERT), SSRIs keep serotonin in the extracellular space where it can continue to bind serotonin receptors. Although an SSRI blocks SERT immediately, antidepressant effects are generally not seen until 2 to 4 weeks of continuous treatment. Over time, increased extracellular availability of serotonin (5-HT) causes $5HT_{1A}$ receptors to become desensitized to serotonin. $5HT_{1A}$ receptors are located on the far end of the presynaptic neuron (not shown, a mile above this page). As desensitization occurs, serotonin stops inhibiting its own release, so serotonin flows more freely from the end of the presynaptic neuron shown below. $5HT_{1A}$ receptor desensitization takes a few weeks, which correlates with onset of therapeutic effect. Anti-inflammatory effects of SSRIs may also contribute. Refer to *Stahl's Essential Psychopharmacology* book for a full visual explanation.

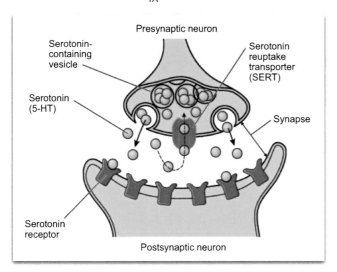

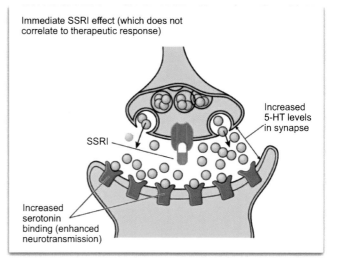

The main side effect leading to patients quitting their SSRI is sexual dysfunction. Unlike TCAs, SSRIs do not cause hypotension or major anticholinergic effects. Other than citalopram (Celexa), SSRIs do not cause significant cardiac conduction delays. SSRIs are initially associated with modest weight loss, which may be followed by modest weight gain with long-term use. SSRIs can cause hyponatremia (low serum sodium) secondary to inappropriate antidiuretic hormone secretion (SIADH) from the pituitary gland.

Rx	SSRI Antidepressant	Interactions	Half–life	Comments
#1	Sertraline (ZOLOFT)	Minimal	26 hr	More likely to cause nausea and diarrhea. OK for first-line
#2	Escitalopram (LEXAPRO)	The fewest interactions of the SSRIs	30 hr	Recommended as first-line SSRI. Fewer side effects and slightly more effective than the other SSRIs.
#3	Citalopram (CELEXA)	Minimal (substrate)	35 hr	QT prolongation if 40 mg dose is exceeded. Choose escitalopram instead.
#4	Fluoxetine (PROZAC)	Strong CYP inhibitor	7 days	More activating. Possible insomnia and appetite suppression. 5-HT discontinuation symptoms less likely thanks to long half-life.
#5	Paroxetine (PAXIL)	Strong CYP inhibitor	20 hr	"More calming". The most sexual side effects, weight gain, sedation, and anticholinergic constipation.
#6	Fluvoxamine (LUVOX)	Very strong CYP inhibitor	16 hr	For OCD only; Lots of kinetic interactions. Short half-life, dosed BID (other SSRIs are QD); Other SSRIs at high doses are similarly effective for OCD.

Uses of SSRIs

- ❖ Depression
- ❖ Anxiety
- ❖ Panic disorder (start low dose)
- ❖ OCD (titrate to high dose)
- ❖ Menopausal hot flashes
- ❖ Somatoform disorders
- ❖ Premature ejaculation
- ❖ Premenstrual dysphoric disorder (PMS)

SSRI risks

- ❖ GI bleed (inhibition of serotonin uptake by platelets)
- ❖ Hyponatremia (low serum sodium)
- ❖ Serotonin syndrome
- ❖ Suicidality (under age 24)
- ❖ Mania, destabilization of bipolar disorder

SSRI side effects

- ❖ Sexual dysfunction (all, especially paroxetine)
- ❖ Modest weight gain with long term use (especially paroxetine)
- ❖ Insomnia (especially fluoxetine)
- ❖ Nausea (short-lived)
- ❖ Diarrhea (sertraline) or constipation (paroxetine)
- ❖ Restlessness / dizziness (short-lived)
- ❖ Bruxism (teeth grinding) which can improve with addition of buspirone (Buspar)

FYI—Medications with the -oxetine suffix:
- ❖ Fluoxetine (Prozac) – SSRI
- ❖ Paroxetine (Paxil) – SSRI
- ❖ Duloxetine (Cymbalta) – SNRI
- ❖ Vortioxetine (Trintellix) – Serotonin modulator & stimulator (SMS)
- ❖ Atomoxetine (Strattera) – Norepinephrine reuptake inhibitor for ADHD

Sertraline (ZOLOFT)
SER tra leen / ZOE loft

"So Soft (on the) Shirt Line"

❖ Antidepressant
❖ Selective serotonin reuptake inhibitor (SSRI)

25
50
100
mg

FDA-approved for:

❖ Major depressive disorder
❖ Obsessive-compulsive disorder
❖ Panic disorder
❖ Post-traumatic stress disorder
❖ Premenstrual dysphoric disorder
❖ Social anxiety disorder

Used off-label for:

❖ Generalized anxiety disorder
❖ Bulimia nervosa
❖ Premature ejaculation

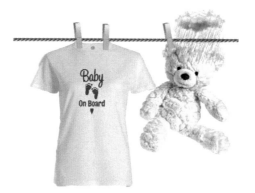

Sertraline is the preferred antidepressant for pregnancy and breastfeeding. Medication exposure to the fetus/baby is minimal.

Ideally, all psychotropic drugs should be avoided from weeks 3 - 10 post-conception, the period of organogenesis. However, untreated depression may be worse for mother and fetus than risk of exposure to most antidepressants..

"Sertraline blocks the serotonin transporter (SERT)" as do all SSRIs. Sertraline (Zoloft) is the #1 prescribed antidepressant and the #14 overall prescribed medication in the United States. It is a reasonable first-line treatment for any of its FDA-approved conditions. Sertraline has no real advantage over escitalopram (Lexapro), which has a slight advantage over sertraline in terms of side effects.

Among SSRIs, sertraline is the most likely to cause diarrhea—*"Zoloft makes your stools So Soft".* "So soft" also refers to sertraline's potential to cause erectile dysfunction, which is a side effect of all SSRIs. In terms of antidepressant-associated sexual dysfunction, sertraline is slightly better than paroxetine (Paxil) and slightly worse than escitalopram.

For any SSRI, treatment of obsessive-compulsive disorder (OCD) may require significantly higher doses than used for depression. Although the FDA max for Zoloft is 200 mg, it may be necessary to go as high as 400 mg for treatment of OCD (titrated gradually).

On drug screens, Zoloft can cause a false positive result for benzodiazepines.

Risk of mortality with single-drug overdose on sertraline is about 1 in 10,000 (Nelson & Spyker, 2017), which is similar to mortality risk of escitalopram.

Zoloft combines well with bupropion (Wellbutrin) for depression with prominent fatigue *("Well-off").* Trazodone (Desyrel) is a common add-on for insomnia. For anxiety, sertraline combines well with buspirone (Buspar) or any benzodiazepine. For bipolar depression or refractory unipolar depression, sertraline can be combined with any mood stabilizer or antipsychotic. Buspirone can counter SSRI-induced sexual dysfunction and bruxism.

Dosing: 50 mg is the starting dose for most indications; FDA max is 200 mg; For treatment of OCD the dose may need to go as high as 400 mg (Stahl, 2016). Taper gradually to avoid unpleasant serotonin discontinuation symptoms.

Information applicable to all SSRIs:

SSRIs block the serotonin reuptake pump. Onset of therapeutic effect is delayed 2–4 weeks. They start working when serotonin $5HT_{1A}$ receptors become desensitized. Some patients experience immediate increased energy or unpleasant restlessness, which is more common with bipolar disorder. Side effects occur sooner than therapeutic effects and often improve over time—nausea, sweating, headache, and bruxism (teeth grinding). Sexual dysfunction is often problematic, and less likely than other side effects to improve with time. SSRIs may increase suicidal thoughts in individuals under age 24.

Following resolution of a single depressive episode, the antidepressant should generally be continued for a year to consolidate recovery. For recurrent episodes, treatment may need to be continued indefinitely. SSRIs are safe and effective for long-term

use, but some patients complain of feeling emotionally flat or "blah", experiencing what has been described as SSRI-Induced Apathy Syndrome. SSRIs may cause a modest weight loss initially, and a modest weight gain with long-term use.

With bipolar individuals, SSRIs may cause "switching" to mania or destabilize mood over time.

When abruptly discontinued, SSRIs may cause serotonin withdrawal symptoms including lightheadedness, "brain zaps", paresthesias, nausea, fatigue and irritability.

SSRIs may decrease serum sodium levels and impair platelet functioning, but risk of significant hyponatremia or bleeding is minimal.

The Zoloft Sad Blob debuted as an advertising mascot in 2001.

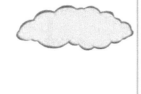

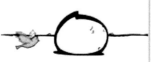

Dynamic interactions:

❖ Serotonergic (strong)
❖ Antiplatelet effect
❖ Hyponatremia

Kinetic interactions:

❖ Although sertraline is a substrate of 2B6 and 2C19, drug interactions involving sertraline are unlikely to be of much clinical significance.
❖ Zoloft is a 2D6 inhibitor when dosed 150 mg or higher, with the potential to modestly increase serum levels of some antipsychotics.

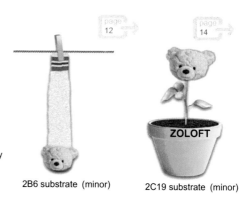

page 12
page 14

2B6 substrate (minor)

2C19 substrate (minor)

#26
2002
$3–$98

Escitalopram (LEXAPRO)
ess sit AL o pram / LEX a pro
"Lexus Pram"

❖ Antidepressant
❖ Selective serotonin
reuptake inhibitor (SSRI)

5
<u>10</u>
20
mg

FDA-approved for:
❖ Major depressive disorder
❖ Generalized anxiety disorder

Used off-label for
❖ Obsessive-compulsive disorder
❖ Post-traumatic stress disorder
❖ Premature ejaculation
❖ Premenstrual dysphoric disorder
❖ Social anxiety disorder
❖ Autism spectrum disorder
❖ Bulimia nervosa

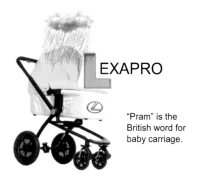

EXAPRO

"Pram" is the British word for baby carriage.

Escitalopram (Lexapro) is the "pure" form of Celexa (citalopram). Escitalopram is the **S**-enantiomer of the molecule, as explained in the citalopram monograph on the following page. Compared to Celexa, Lexapro is safer, often better tolerated, and possibly more effective. There is <u>no reason to choose citalopram over escitalopram</u>—"*S-citalopram is Superior to racemic citalopram*".

<u>S</u> for "<u>S</u>inister" = <u>L</u> for <u>L</u>eft-handed enantiomer

Escitalopram is the <u>best choice for a first-line</u> antidepressant. It is <u>the most selective</u> inhibitor of the serotonin pump among all SSRIs. Several clinical trials and meta-analyses indicate escitalopram may be <u>slightly more effective</u> than other SSRIs. Escitalopram has an allosteric effect at the serotonin transporter that distinguishes it from other SSRIs. 10 mg of escitalopram is predictably <u>more</u> effective than 20 mg of citalopram (which contains 10 mg escitalopram and 10 mg R-citalopram).

Lexapro has the <u>fewest side effects</u> of all the SSRIs. At the starting dose of 10 mg, side effects are comparable to placebo. It is unlikely to cause weight gain or sedation. It has minimal drug-drug interactions. Lexapro is <u>safe</u>. Risk of mortality with single-drug overdose on escitalopram is about 1 in 9,000 (Nelson & Spyker, 2017).

For depression, escitalopram is at least as effective as SNRI antidepressants. Although venlafaxine (Effexor) and duloxetine (Cymbalta) have the additional mechanism of blocking the norepinephrine transporter, do not expect either of them to outperform Lexapro.

Although escitalopram may be the overall winner among SSRIs, with all psychotropic drugs there is marked inter-individual variability in tolerability and therapeutic response. If an individual is doing wonderfully on another antidepressant, there is usually no reason to change to escitalopram.

Escitalopram is regarded as safe for pregnancy and breastfeeding, but sertraline (Zoloft) is safer.

Serum levels of escitalopram peak about 5 hours after ingestion. Half-life is around 30 hours, so steady-state concentration should be achieved within 7 days. Upon discontinuation, escitalopram should be cleared from the body within 7 days.

Dosing: Start escitalopram <u>10 mg</u> QD (AM or PM), after meals for the first few days, then with or without food. May increase to <u>20 mg</u> in one week, but generally you would wait about 4 weeks to see if it is necessary to advance the dose. Although the FDA max for Lexapro is 20 mg, it is not unusual to see it prescribed up to 30 mg for major depression. It can be safely dosed up to 60 mg daily for OCD (Stahl, 2016). <u>When converting from citalopram (Celexa), use half the milligram dose of escitalopram</u>. 20 mg of Lexapro is predictable more effective than 40 mg of Celexa. Use a lower dose for elderly individuals because serum levels will be about 50% higher. If the patient is taking omeprazole (Prilosec) or esomeprazole (Nexium), consider starting escitalopram at 5 mg. Renal impairment: no adjustment needed. Hepatic impairment: consider lower dose. Taper to discontinue to avoid unpleasant serotonin withdrawal symptoms.

Dynamic interactions:
❖ Serotonergic (strong)
❖ QT prolongation (minimal)
❖ Antiplatelet effect
❖ Hyponatremia

Kinetic interactions:
❖ Fewer interactions than most SSRIs
❖ As a 2C19 substrate, escitalopram levels are increased by **proton pump inhibitors** (PPIs). Avoid omeprazole (Prilosec) and and esomeprazole (Nexium), which increase escitalopram levels by 80–90%. Instead, choose pantoprazole (Protonix) or lansoprazole (Prevacid), which only increase escitalopram by about 20%. Although more expensive, rabeprazole (Aciphex) does not affect escitalopram levels.

page 14 →

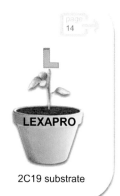

LEXAPRO

2C19 substrate

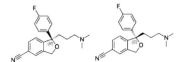

#21
1998
$2–$35

Citalopram (CELEXA)
si TAL o pram / SEL ex a

"Sell Lexus Pram"

❖ Antidepressant
❖ Selective serotonin
  reuptake inhibitor (SSRI)

10
20
40
mg

FDA-approved for:

❖ Major depressive disorder

Used off-label for

❖ Generalized anxiety disorder
❖ Social anxiety disorder
❖ Post-traumatic stress disorder
❖ Premature ejaculation
❖ Premenstrual dysphoric disorder
❖ Autism spectrum disorder
❖ Bulimia nervosa

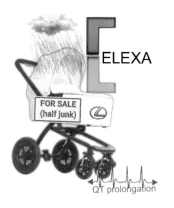

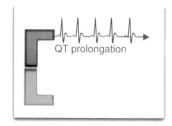

page 41 →

Celexa is a combo of: S-citalopram   = the active Left-handed molecule (available as Lexapro),

and its mirror image molecule: R-citalopram: R-citalopram   = "Rubbish" Right-handed molecule, in a 50/50 ratio

Citalopram (Celexa) is the old 50% pure version of escitalopram (Lexapro). 50% of Celexa is the right-handed enantiomer R-citalopram. S-citalopram is the most selective (for serotonin reuptake inhibition) of all SSRIs. R-citalopram is ineffective and causes QT interval prolongation.

The plasma concentration of S-citalopram (escitalopram) is usually one third of the total citalopram concentration, with the implication that the other two thirds of the total citalopram concentration is inactive as an antidepressant (Burke & Kratochvil, 2002).

In 2012 the FDA released a warning for QT prolongation with Celexa and reduced the maximum approved dose from 60 mg to 40 mg. Lexapro does not have this warning. The warning may have been unwarranted, because rates of sudden unexpected death with high-dose citalopram is no higher than with other high-dose SSRIs (Ray et al, 2017). When VA patients were taken off citalopram because of the FDA warning, rates of depression increased and incidents of arrhythmias were not affected (Rector et al, 2016).

Although rarely clinically significant, QT prolongation by R-citalopram poses some risk in overdose situations. Although the risk of single-drug overdose death with Celexa is only about 1 in 1,850, mortality risk is over 4x higher than with Lexapro. QT prolongation by Celexa could potentially be risky when it is prescribed along with other QT-prolonging medications.

Celexa 20 mg is roughly equivalent to Lexapro 10 mg, as would be expected, given that half of Celexa is junk. Even at double the milligram dose, Celexa is predictably less effective than Lexapro. L-citalopram has an allosteric effect at the serotonin transporter that R-citalopram interferes with.

For initiation of antidepressant treatment, there is no reason to choose Celexa over Lexapro. So, why is anyone on citalopram? Many patients are on Celexa because, when their medication was started, Lexapro was more expensive. Celexa has been available generically since 2004. Lexapro went generic in 2012. When a drug goes off patent, it generally takes several years for enough manufacturers to enter the market for the drug to become dirt cheap.

Of the other SSRIs, paroxetine (Paxil) and sertraline (Zoloft) have always been pure enantiomers. Fluvoxamine (Luvox) lacks a chiral center, so a mirror image molecule does not exist. Fluoxetine (Prozac) is a racemic mixture, but R-fluoxetine and L-fluoxetine inhibit serotonin reuptake equally.

Bottom line: If starting an SSRI, choose escitalopram rather than citalopram. If a patient already established on citalopram is doing wonderfully, "don't try to fix what ain't broken".

Dosing: Celexa is started at 20 mg QD, dosed in AM or PM. In about 4 weeks may increase to FDA maximum of 40 mg. If higher strength is needed, change to Lexapro 20 mg, which is predictable more effective than Celexa 40 mg.

Dynamic interactions:

❖ Serotonergic (strong)
❖ QT prolongation (moderate)
❖ Antiplatelet effect
❖ Hyponatremia

Kinetic interactions:

❖ 2C19 substrate
❖ 2C19 poor metabolizers should not
  exceed 20 mg of citalopram
❖ See escitalopram monograph for preferred
  proton pump inhibitors (2C19 inHibitors)

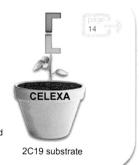

page 14 →

CELEXA

2C19 substrate

Fluoxetine (PROZAC)
flu OX e teen / PRO zak
"Prolonged sack of the Flustered ox"

#29
1987
$2–$36

❖ Antidepressant
❖ Selective serotonin reuptake inhibitor (SSRI)

10
20
40
mg

FDA-approved for:
❖ Major depressive disorder
❖ Obsessive-compulsive disorder
❖ Bulimia nervosa
❖ Panic disorder
❖ Premenstrual dysphoric disorder (Sarafem brand)

Used off-label for:
❖ Other anxiety disorders
❖ Premature ejaculation (to Prolong intercouse)
❖ Binge eating disorder

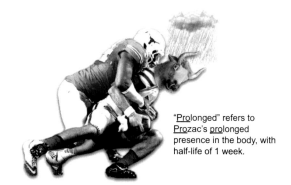

"Prolonged" refers to Prozac's prolonged presence in the body, with half-life of 1 week.

Fluoxetine (Prozac) was the first available SSRI, released to the US market in 1987. Among antidepressants, Prozac has the best evidence for treatment of depression among children and adolescents. It is the only FDA-approved medication for treatment of depression in children (age 8 and older).

For adults, Lexapro and Zoloft are generally preferred because Prozac interacts with numerous medications. Specifically, Prozac is an inHibitor of several CYP enzymes. If Prozac were a newly introduced drug, it would be unlikely to receive FDA approval due to the magnitude of these interactions.

Among SSRIs, Prozac is considered the most activating/energizing (as opposed to calming). As a result it is more likely to cause anxiety and insomnia than other SSRIs. It is safe for those with sleep apnea because it is a respiratory stimulant. It is not expected to cause weight gain and may result in modest weight loss. As with other SSRIs, the most troublesome side effect is sexual dysfunction.

Prozac has a very long elimination half-life of about 7 days. In other words, Prozac has a Prolonged presence in your body. A mnemonic from Dr. Jonathan Heldt's book Memorable Psychopharmacology compares the half-life of fluoxetine to the 7 days its takes to recover from the flu (influenza).

With chronic use, fluoxetine is detectable in the body up to five weeks after discontinuation (elimination half-life x 5). Since Prozac "tapers itself" off over weeks when stopped abruptly, there should be no serotonin withdrawal symptoms. Thanks to long half-life, missed doses are of less consequence (compared to antidepressants with shorter half-lives). If the patient forgets to take a dose on Monday, it is OK to take a double dose on Tuesday. This would not be advisable with most other psychotropics.

Fluoxetine is safe. Risk of death with single-drug overdose is no more than 1 in 10,000.

SYMBYAX is a fixed dose combination of fluoxetine with the antipsychotic olanzapine (Zyprexa), approved for acute depressive episodes of bipolar I disorder and for treatment-resistant major depression. Released in 2003, Symbyax (mnemonic Symbiotic Ox) was marketed heavily to primary care physicians, who likely underestimated olanzapine's potential for causing weight gain and diabetes. The fixed doses of olanzapine/fluoxetine in Symbyax are 3/25mg, 6/25 mg, 6/50 mg, and 12/50 mg taken in the evening.

For the sake of trivia, there exists a 90 mg fluoxetine ER capsule intended for once weekly dosing called PROZAC WEEKLY. It runs $50 per capsule. That's $200 monthly, compared to $4–$10 for a month of generic QD fluoxetine.

When discontinuing fluoxetine 40 mg or less, it may be ok just to stop without tapering, thanks to is long half-life. However, some patients may need a hyperbolic taper as described on page 58. To come off of higher doses, you will want to taper over several months. Switching from fluoxetine to another antidepressant can be tricky due to fluoxetine's long half-life. When switching to another modern serotonergic antidepressant, consider a washout period before starting the new antidepressant. The risk of serotonin syndrome is minimal with some overlap of two SSRIs (or an SSRI and an SNRI), so you do not have to wait for fluoxetine to be entirely cleared by the body. However, when switching from fluoxetine to an MAOI, there can be no overlap, because serotonin syndrome is a major risk. You need to wait at least five weeks after stopping fluoxetine to start the MAOI. For the other SSRIs, you only have to wait 2 weeks to start the MAOI.

Dosing:

Fluoxetine, available in 10 mg, 20 mg, and 40 mg capsules, is typically started (for adults) at 20 mg QD. It can be titrated in 20 mg increments to the FDA max dose of 80 mg QD. As a rule of thumb, you would want to wait about 4 weeks between dose increases. If there is a prior effective dose (for a particular patient) you are targeting, you can titrate faster. See above for discontinuation strategies.

For obsessive-compulsive disorder (OCD), you can go as high as 120 mg daily (Stahl, 2016). OCD often requires heroically high doses of SSRIs, and fluoxetine is a safe option.

For premenstrual dysphoric disorder (PMDD), you can take 20 mg QD starting 14 days prior to the anticipated onset of menses through the first full day of menstruation and repeating with each cycle. The brand SARAFEM (10 mg, 20 mg) is FDA-approved for this indication, but you will want to prescribe generic fluoxetine. For PMDD there is no proven benefit in exceeding 20 mg/day.

The "fluffers" - infamous inHibitors of CYP enzymes:

❖ Fluvoxamine (Luvox)
❖ Fluoxetine (Prozac)
❖ Fluconazole (Diflucan)

Fluoxetine is a less potent enzyme inhibitor than the other two.

Dynamic interactions:
❖ Serotonergic (strong)
❖ Antiplatelet effect
❖ Hyponatremia

Kinetic interactions:
❖ Fluoxetine is an inHibitor of 2D6 and 2C19. This results in numerous interactions that markedly increase blood levels of various victim drugs (substrates).
❖ Although fluoxetine itself is a 2D6 and 2C9 substrate, clinically significant victimization is not expected.

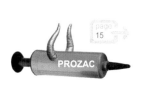

2D6 inHibitor (strong)

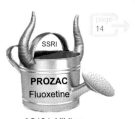

2C19 inHibitor (moderate)

Paroxetine (PAXIL)
par OX e tine / PAX il

"Pear rocks a teen (Paxil Rose)"

❖ Antidepressant
❖ Selective serotonin reuptake inhibitor (SSRI)

ER	
12.5	10
25	20
37.5	30
mg	40
	mg

FDA-approved for:

❖ Major depressive disorder
❖ Obsessive-compulsive disorder
❖ Generalized anxiety disorder
❖ Panic disorder
❖ Social anxiety
❖ Post-traumatic stress disorder
❖ Menopausal vasomotor symptoms (hot flashes) at low 7.5 mg strength branded as BRISDELLE

Used off-label for:

❖ Premenstrual dysphoric disorder
❖ Premature ejaculation

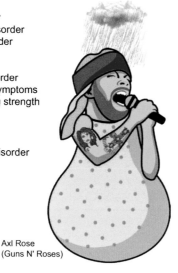

Axl Rose
(Guns N' Roses)

Paroxetine (Paxil) has the reputation as a calming (as opposed to energizing) antidepressant. However, there are several reasons to choose a different SSRI. Although paroxetine is FDA-approved for more anxious conditions than other SSRIs, it has performed no better for anxiety in head-to-head trials (Sanchez et al, 2014).

Disadvantages of paroxetine compared to other SSRIs:

► More fatigue
► More weight gain
► More sexual dysfunction
► More likely to cause withdrawal symptoms with missed doses
► More CYP interactions (excluding fluvoxamine)
► More anticholinergic effects
► Risk of dementia (anticholinergic), unlike other SSRIs
► Risk of birth defects
► Less effective than escitalopram, even for anxiety disorders

Axl Rose has short stature. Among antidepressants, Paxil has a relatively short elimination half-life of 21 hours. A missed dose may result in unpleasant serotonin withdrawal symptoms.

Paroxetine is the only SSRI with significant anticholinergic effects, making it a bad SSRI choice for elderly individuals. As a result of this anticholinergic activity, Paxil is the most constipating SSRI—"Paxil packs it in". Paroxetine is the most likely SSRI to cause tachycardia, which is an anticholinergic effect. Prolonged exposure to anticholinergic medications is a risk factor for cognitive decline. Paxil is the only SSRI associated with increased risk (2-fold) of developing dementia (Heath et al, 2018).

Paroxetine has more potential to cause fatigue and weight gain than other modern antidepressants, but less so than some TCAs.

All SSRIs commonly decrease sexual desire, disrupt the sexual pleasure response, and increase latency to orgasm. Among SSRIs, Paxil is the most likely to cause sexual dysfunction. Since Paxil is the "best" at interfering with orgasms, it is the SSRI of choice for off-label treatment of premature ejaculation. Its short half-life makes it handy as a PRN for this purpose.

There may be a possibility of birth defects if Paxil is taken in early pregnancy. Under pre-2015 FDA pregnancy risk categories, paroxetine was pregnancy Category D, while other SSRIs were Category C.

As a strong 2D6 inhibitor, paroxetine is more likely to cause problematic drug-drug interactions than the other commonly used SSRIs. Fluvoxamine (Luvox), a stronger inhibitor of CYP enzymes, is worse than Paxil in terms of interactions.

The enteric coated controlled-release formulation of paroxetine, Paxil CR, is less likely to cause nausea. Nausea is a short-lived side effect, and after the first week the CR formulation offers little advantage over immediate-release paroxetine.

Dosing: Start 20 mg AM. Depending on the indication, FDA max is 50–60 mg. For OCD start 20 mg AM, increase by 10 mg weekly to target of at least 40 mg. FDA max for OCD is 60 mg, but can go as high as 100 mg (Stahl, 2016). The target dose for panic disorder is 40 mg. Consider twice daily dosing ≥ 40 mg. For menopausal hot flashes, rather than using expensive 7.5 mg paroxetine (Brisdelle), prescribe 10 mg generic paroxetine HS. Taper gradually to discontinue to avoid serotonin withdrawal symptoms.

Among SSRIs, Paxil has a relatively short half-life of 21 hours.

short

Signs of serotonin discontinuation include:

page 58

► Lightheadedness
► Paresthesias
► Nausea
► Fatigue
► Irritability

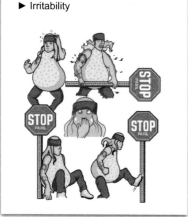

Dynamic interactions:
❖ Serotonergic (strong)
❖ Antiplatelet effect
❖ Hyponatremia

Kinetic interactions:
❖ 2C9 inHibitor (moderate)
❖ 2D6 inHibitor (strong)
❖ 2D6 substrate

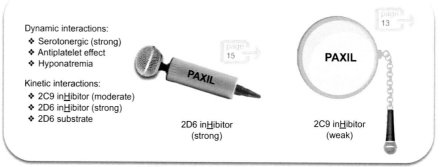

page 15
page 13

2D6 inHibitor (strong)

PAXIL

2C9 inHibitor (weak)

1996
$20–$120

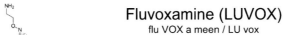

Fluvoxamine (LUVOX)
flu VOX a meen / LU vox

"Glove-ox"

❖ Selective serotonin reuptake inhibitor (SSRI)
❖ OCD medication
❖ Potent CYP in**H**ibitor

25
50
100
mg

FDA-approved for:

❖ Obsessive-compulsive disorder (OCD)

Used off-label for:

❖ Social anxiety disorder (rarely)
❖ Strategic in**H**ibition of CYP1A2 with clozapine as described on page 11
❖ Premature ejaculation

Fluvoxamine (Luvox) is an SSRI approved exclusively for OCD, a disorder characterized by obsessions (recurrent intrusive thoughts) that the individual may attempt to neutralize with a compulsive repetitive behavior or ritual, e.g., flicking a light switch 50 times.

Three other SSRIs are FDA-approved for OCD—fluoxetine (Prozac), paroxetine (Paxil), and sertraline (Zoloft). Off-label, escitalopram (Lexapro) at high dose may be a better choice than fluvoxamine for OCD because it highly selective for blocking serotonin transporters and has fewer side effects.

✱ Although not used for depression, fluvoxamine is properly referred to as an antidepressant.

Luvox is a potent in**H**ibitor of multiple CYP enzymes, causing increased serum levels of many co-administered medications. CYP1A2 inhibition by fluvoxamine can be used for strategic advantage in combination with clozapine (Clozaril) as explained on page 11.

50 mg HS is the starting fluvoxamine dose for the first week, then 50 mg BID. Envision the mascot flicking a light switch 50 times. Additional dose increases will likely be necessary for fluvoxamine to be effective for OCD. With any SSRI, effective treatment of OCD demands a high dose, often exceeding the FDA max.

Fluvoxamine should be dosed BID for maintenance because it has the shortest half-life of all available SSRIs (15 hours). Other SSRIs are generally dosed once daily.

Among SSRIs, fluvoxamine is the least likely to cause sexual dysfunction (La Torre et al, 2013), although > 50% of patients are still affected. Owing to short half-life, fluvoxamine is a reasonable PRN treatment for premature ejaculation.

Dosing: For OCD start 50 mg HS, then increase to 50 mg BID in 4–7 days. May increase by 50 mg/day every 4–7 days. FDA maximum is 300 mg/day but may go as high as 450 mg (Stahl, 2016) in divided doses. Dosing is similar for social anxiety disorder. Taper gradually to discontinue.

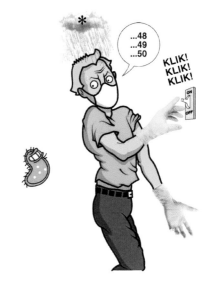

...48
...49
...50

KLIK!
KLIK!
KLIK!

Serotonergic medications need to be prescribed at high dose to effectively treat obsessive-compulsive disorder.

*Escitalopram is used off-label for OCD.

Serotonergic med	Class	FDA max	Max for OCD (Stahl, 2016)
Clomipramine (Anafranil)	TCA	250 mg	250 mg
Fluvoxamine (Luvox)	SSRI	300 mg	450 mg
Escitalopram (Lexapro)*	SSRI	20 mg	60 mg
Fluoxetine (Prozac)	SSRI	80 mg	120 mg
Paroxetine (Paxil)	SSRI	60 mg	100 mg
Sertraline (Zoloft)	SSRI	200 mg	400 mg

Due to short half-life, serotonin discontinuation symptoms are common if Luvox is stopped abruptly:

► Lightheadedness
► Paresthesias
► Nausea
► Fatigue
► Irritability

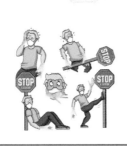

For maintenance, Luvox is dosed BID because it has the shortest half-life among SSRIs (15 hr).

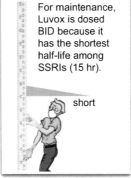

short

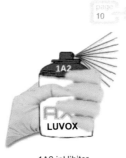

Dynamic interactions:

❖ Serotonergic (strong)
❖ Antiplatelet effect
❖ Hyponatremia

Kinetic interactions:

❖ Luvox is a "fluffer", i.e., in**H**ibitor of several CYP enzymes. This results in numerous drug-drug interactions causing the serum level of the victim drug (substrate) to increase markedly
❖ Ramelteon (Rozerem) is contraindicated because ramelteon levels increase 100-fold! (1A2)
❖ Tizanidine (Zanaflex) is contraindicated because tizanidine levels increase 10-fold (1A2)
❖ Pimozide (Orap) is contraindicated (3A4)
❖ Although fluvoxamine Itself is a 2D6 and 1A2 substrate, clinically significant victimization is not expected

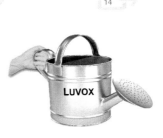

1A2 in**H**ibitor (strong)

2C19 in**H**ibitor (strong)

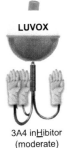

LUVOX

3A4 in**H**ibitor (moderate)

Serotonin-norepinephrine reuptake inhibitors (SNRIs)

SNRIs increase the extracellular availability of neurotransmitters serotonin (5-HT) and norepinephrine (NE).
Think of serotonin as calming ("serene") and norepinephrine (NE), also known as noradrenalin, as eNErgizing.

SNRI Antidepressant	U.S. Market	Uses	Comments
Duloxetine (CYMBALTA)	2004	Depression, Fibromyalgia, Neuropathic pain, Anxiety	Duloxetine is involved in more CYP interactions, than the other SNRIs.
Venlafaxine (EFFEXOR)	1994	Depression, Anxiety, Chronic pain	More dangerous in overdose than other SNRIs
Desvenlafaxine (PRISTIQ)	2007	Depression	Less effective and more side effects than Effexor XR.
Milnacipran (SAVELLA)	2009	Fibromyalgia	Titration pack 12.5 mg (#5), 25 mg (#8), 50 mg (#42)
Levomilnacipran (FETZIMA)	2013	Depression	L-enantiomer of milnacipran (Savella)

Some tricyclic antidepressants (TCAs) are SNRIs by mechanism, although TCAs also block off-target receptors (acetylcholine, histamine, alpha-1).

TCA Antidepressant	U.S. Market	Uses	Comments
Amitriptyline (ELAVIL)	1961	Depression, Neuropathic pain, Migraine prophylaxis, Fibromyalgia, Postherpetic neuralgia, Insomnia	5-HT > NE More sedating than newer SNRIs; Also 5-HT$_2$ receptor antagonist
Doxepin (SINEQUAN, SILENOR)	1969	Depression, Insomnia	Sedating at low dose due antihistamine properties; NE > 5-HT at higher doses; Also 5-HT$_2$ receptor antagonist
Clomipramine (ANAFRANIL)	1990	Obsessive-compulsive disorder (OCD)	5-HT > > NE
Imipramine (TOFRANIL)	1957	Depression	5-HT > NE
Amoxapine (ASENDIN)	1992	Depression	NE > 5-HT, Antipsychotic properties due to D2 antagonism

SNRIs that are not classified as antidepressants:

Other SNRIs	U.S. Market	Uses	Comments
Tramadol (ULTRAM)	1995	Pain	Weak opioid also; Schedule IV controlled substance
Sibutramine (MERIDIA)	1997–2010	Obesity	Removed from market in 2010 due to risk heart attack and stroke

"Atypical Antidepressants"
Newer antidepressants not classified as TCAs, MAOIs, SSRIs, or SNRIs

Atypical antidepressant	Class	Abbrev	Cost/mo	
Nefazodone (SERZONE)	Serotonin Antagonist & Reuptake Inhibitor	SARI	$68	Developed as a non-sedating variant of trazodone. Rarely prescribed. Rare occurrence of severe liver damage.
Trazodone (DESYREL)		SARI	$4	Widely prescribed at low dose, solely as a sleep medication
Mirtazapine (REMERON)	Noradrenergic & Specific Serotonergic Antidepressant	NaSSA	$11	Great for sleep and appetite stimulation, more so at lower dose. At higher dose, noradrenergic (NE) activity is more prominent.
Bupropion (WELLBUTRIN)	Norepinephrine & Dopamine Reuptake Inhibitor	NDRI	$25	Like a mild stimulant—helpful for ADHD, appetite suppression and smoking cessation. Improves sexual functioning. Seizures at high dose.
Vilazodone (VIIBRYD)	Serotonin Modulator & Stimulator	SMS	$200	"Hybrid" of SSRI & 5-HT$_{1A}$ partial agonist. Mechanism of action is like a combo of an SSRI and the anxiolytic buspirone (Buspar).
Vortioxetine (TRINTELLIX)		SMS	$300	Serotonin reuptake inhibitor, 5-HT$_{1A}$ agonist, 5-HT$_{1B}$ partial agonist, 5-HT$_3$ antagonist & 5-HT$_7$ antagonist.

Duloxetine (CYMBALTA)

du LOX e tine / cym BAL ta

"Dueling Cymbals"

#48
2004
$6–$166

❖ Antidepressant
❖ Serotonin-norepinephrine reuptake inhibitor (SNRI)
❖ 5-HT > NE

20
30
40
60
mg

FDA-approved for:

❖ Major depressive disorder
❖ Generalized anxiety disorder
❖ Diabetic neuropathy
❖ Fibromyalgia
❖ Chronic musculoskeletal pain

Used off-label for:

❖ Stress urinary incontinence
❖ ADHD

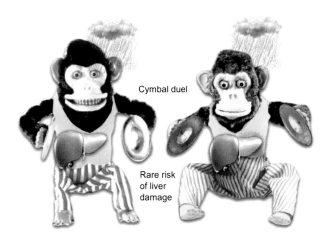

Cymbal duel

Rare risk of liver damage

The SNRI duloxetine (Cymbalta) is reasonable first-line choice for depressed patients with comorbid pain syndromes. Among antidepressants, it stands out as being <u>particularly effective for generalized anxiety disorder</u> (GAD).

Side effects may include <u>nausea</u> (22%), dry mouth (16%), fatigue (11%), dizziness (11%), somnolence, constipation, diarrhea, insomnia, agitation, sweating, headaches, and sexual dysfunction. Duloxetine is <u>not expected to cause appreciable weight gain</u>. Hypertension (1%) due to duloxetine does not appear to be dose-dependent. The discontinuation rate of duloxetine due to side effects was 15% (versus 5% for placebo).

Compared to the SNRI venlafaxine (Effexor), duloxetine is more likely to cause <u>nausea</u> but less likely to elevate blood pressure. Duloxetine is less likely than venlafaxine to cause serotonin withdrawal symptoms upon discontinuation.

Duloxetine is more likely to be involved in clinically significant CYP interactions than venlafaxine.

<u>Serious liver damage</u> is possible with duloxetine, although <u>rare</u>. It is not considered necessary to closely monitor liver enzymes (beyond routine screening labs for all patients).

<u>Avoid prescribing duloxetine to alcoholics or those with known liver problems</u>.

Risk of death from a single-drug overdose with duloxetine is about 1 in 3,500, making it safer than venlafaxine (1 in 800).

Peak plasma levels are achieved at 3 hours. Half-life is 12 hours, so steady-state concentrations are achieved within 3 days of oral dosing (5 x 12 hours). Upon discontinuation, duloxetine is cleared from the body within 3 days (also 5 x 12 hours) and there are no active metabolites.

<u>For depression, the FDA maximum of 120 mg was found no more effective than 60 mg</u>. For pain, the 120 mg dose (divided 60 mg BID) can be more effective.

Dosing: Duloxetine can be dosed BID or QD, either AM or HS. Consider starting 30 mg QD x 1 wk, then increase to target dose of <u>60 mg QD</u> or 30 mg BID. For depression, the FDA maximum of 120 mg is rarely more effective than 60 mg. Doses over 60 mg may be more effective for pain. 120 mg dose is usually divided to 60 mg BID. Taper gradually to discontinue to avoid serotonin withdrawal symptoms.

Dynamic interactions:

❖ Serotonergic
❖ Antiplatelet effect
❖ Hyponatremia
❖ Hy<u>p</u>ertension

Kinetic interactions:

❖ 2D6 in<u>H</u>ibitor (moderate)
❖ 1A2 substrate
 – decreased 30% by smoking
 – increased 3-fold by fluvoxamine (Luvox)
❖ 2D6 substrate

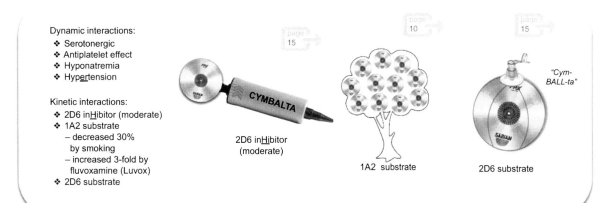

2D6 in<u>H</u>ibitor (moderate)

1A2 substrate

"Cym-BALL-ta"

2D6 substrate

page 15

page 10

page 15

#51
1995
$6–$105

Venlafaxine (EFFEXOR)
ven la FAX ine / e FEX er

"Vanilla faxing (eFax'er)"

❖ Antidepressant
❖ Serotonin-norepinephrine reuptake inhibitor (SNRI)
❖ 5-HT > NE

XR 37.5
75
150
mg

FDA-approved for:

❖ Major depressive disorder
❖ Generalized anxiety disorder
❖ Social anxiety disorder
❖ Panic disorder

Used off-label for:

❖ ADHD
❖ Migraine prophylaxis
❖ Post-traumatic stress disorder
❖ Fibromyalgia
❖ Cataplexy
❖ Vasomotor symptoms of menopause
❖ Premenstrual dysphoric disorder

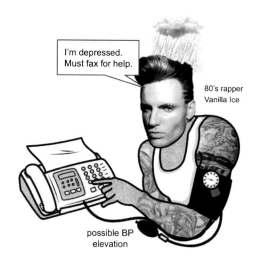

I'm depressed. Must fax for help.

80's rapper
Vanilla Ice

possible BP elevation

The SNRI venlafaxine (Effexor) is a reasonable second-line antidepressant, potentially first-line for depressed individuals suffering from chronic pain. Effexor XR and duloxetine (Cymbalta) are equally popular SNRIs, #51 and #48 most prescribed medications in the US, respectively.

When Effexor was introduced in 1995 prescribers nicknamed it "Side-Effexor" due to nausea and fatigue. Effexor XR (extended-release) was introduced in 1998 and became widely prescribed because it is much better tolerated. Choose the XR formulation, which is also less expensive than the rarely prescribed immediate-release venlafaxine. The only scenario when immediate-release Effexor is preferred is with bariatric surgery patients. For either formulation of Effexor, it is recommended to take it with food to minimize nausea.

Peak plasma concentrations are achieved within 2 to 3 hours for the IR formulation and within 5.5 hours for the XR formulation.

Effexor acts as an SSRI at low doses (37.5 mg, 75 mg) and an SNRI at higher doses (150 mg plus). 75 mg/day is the minimum effective dose for treatment of depression

Venlafaxine has a short half-life of 5 hours, and the half-life of the active metabolite O-desmethylvenlafaxine (ODV) is 11 hours. ODV is available as the antidepressant desvenlafaxine (Pristiq), which appears to be less effective than Effexor for depression.

Incidence of blood pressure elevation with the XR formulation is 1%. With the IR formulation, incidence of hypertension is about 5%, and as high as 13% at doses exceeding 300 mg.

In addition to raising blood pressure, venlafaxine may induce seizures in overdose, making it the most dangerous modern antidepressant (non-TCA, non-MAOI). Risk of single-drug overdose death with venlafaxine is about 1 in 839.

For depression, venlafaxine is no more effective than the SSRI escitalopram (Lexapro), which has fewer side effects. For generalized anxiety disorder, venlafaxine is more effective than buspirone (Buspar).

Venlafaxine can cause false positives for PCP on drug tests.

FDA max is 225 mg, but for severe depression 300 mg may be more effective. Take caution because blood pressure elevation is dose dependent. Taper off Effexor slowly to avoid symptoms of serotonin withdrawal syndrome.

XR Dosing: Specify the extended-release formulation Effexor XR, (venlafaxine ER) except for in bariatric surgery patients. Start Effexor XR 37.5 or 75 mg QD with food (to ameliorate nausea), with target of 150–225 mg QD. FDA max is 225 mg, but 300 mg may be more effective for depression. For treatment of pain the dose can go as high as high as 450 mg/day if blood pressure is monitored closely. May increase in 75 mg increments every 4–7 days.

IR dosing: For bariatric surgery patients, prescribe venlafaxine IR which is available in 25, 37.5, 50, 75, and 100 mg tablets, given in divided doses BID or TID. The FDA maximum for IR venlafaxine is 375 mg/day in divided doses (125 mg TID).

Signs of serotonin discontinuation include:

page 58

❖ Lightheadedness
❖ Paresthesias
❖ Nausea
❖ Fatigue
❖ Irritability

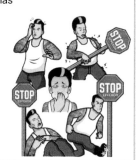

Effexor XR

37.5 mg	75 mg	150 mg
"SSRI"	"SSRI"	SNRI

Effexor acts as an SSRI at low doses (37.5 mg, 75 mg) and an SNRI at higher doses (150 mg plus).

Dynamic interactions:

❖ Serotonergic
❖ Antiplatelet effect
❖ Hyponatremia
❖ Hypertension

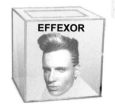

EFFEXOR

page 18

Kinetic interactions:

❖ 2D6 converts venlafaxine to an active metabolite (desvenlafaxine). 2D6 metabolizer phenotype does not affect efficacy, although Individuals with 2D6 poor metabolizer genotype may experience more side effects.
❖ Also a substrate of 2C19 and 3A4 substrate
❖ Kinetic interactions occur but are unlikely to be clinically relevant—"in a box".

Cafer's Psychopharmacology | cafermed.com

Desvenlafaxine (PRISTIQ)
des ven la FAX ine / Pris TIQ

"Desk faxing Pressed steak"

- ❖ Antidepressant
- ❖ Serotonin-norepinephrine reuptake inhibitor (SNRI)
- ❖ 5-HT > NE

25
50
100
mg

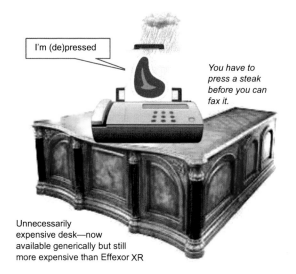

I'm (de)pressed

You have to press a steak before you can fax it.

Unnecessarily expensive desk—now available generically but still more expensive than Effexor XR

Pill formulations with "ghost pill" shells passing in feces:

Sources include:
Tungaraza et al, 2003

Antipsychotics
 Invega (paliperidone ER)
Antidepressants
 Wellbutrin XL (bupropion XL)
 Effexor XR (venlafaxine ER)
 Pristiq (desvenlafaxine ER)
Stimulants
 Concerta (methylphenidate ER)
 Ritalin SR (methylphenidate SR)
 Focalin XR (dexmethylphenidate ER)
Mood Stabilizer
 Tegretol XR (carbamazepine ER)
Opioid
 Oxycontin (oxycodone ER)
 Exalgo (hydromorphone ER)

FDA-approved for:
- ❖ Major depressive disorder

Used off-label for:
- ❖ Same as venlafaxine (Effexor)

Desvenlafaxine (Pristiq), also known as O-desmethy-venlafaxine (ODV), is an <u>active metabolite of venlafaxine</u> (Effexor). Pristiq was introduced to the US market in 2007, thirteen years after the release of Effexor. The European Union did not approve Pristiq because it is probably <u>less effective than Effexor</u> and has no clear advantage over Effexor.

Pristiq is one of the few antidepressants visualized in a bubble, to signify that kinetic interactions are highly unlikely. Pristiq is subject to fewer kinetic interactions than Effexor, but Effexor has relatively low potential for clinically significant interactions anyhow (visualized in a box).

All desvenlafaxine (Pristiq) tablets are extended-release (ER), so you don't have to write "ER" on a desvenlafaxine script. To get ER venlafaxine (page 48) you have to specify "Effexor XR" or "venlafaxine ER".

Dosing: <u>50 mg QD</u> is the only recommended dose. The 100 mg dose adds no benefit, and is more likely to cause nausea. The FDA max is 400 mg, although this is considered too high.

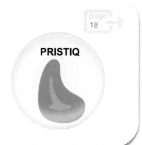

Dynamic interactions:
- ❖ Serotonergic
- ❖ Antiplatelet effect
- ❖ Hyponatremia
- ❖ Hypertension

Kinetic interactions:
- ❖ Minimal potential for clinically relevant pharmacokinetic interactions - "in a bubble"

page 18 →

PRISTIQ

Desvenlafaxine (KHEDEZLA)
des ven la FAX ine / kah DEZ la

"Desk faxing on Kid's desk"

- ❖ Antidepressant
- ❖ Serotonin-norepinephrine reuptake inhibitor (SNRI)
- ❖ 5-HT > NE

50
100
mg

FDA-approved for:
- ❖ Major depressive disorder (adults)

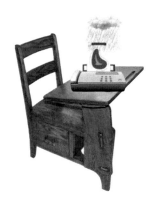

Desvenlafaxine is also available as the brand name Khedezla (released 2014) which is <u>equivalent to Pristiq</u> (2007). Both Pristiq and Khedezla are extended-release (ER) formulations of desvenlafaxine, both indicated for major depressive disorder, both dosed once daily. Pristiq is a succinate salt with a half-life of 10.4 hours, while Khedezla is a base with a half-life of 10.6 hours.

The approval of Khedezla was based on the original Pristiq efficacy studies.

Studies have found desvenlafaxine to be ineffective for children with depression (Weihs et al, 2017). *"Kid's desk ain't for kids."*

Desvenlafaxine has been available generically since 2017.

Dosing: Same as Pristiq

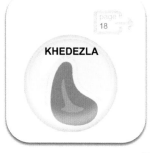

page 18 →

KHEDEZLA

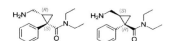

Milnacipran (SAVELLA)

mil NA si pran / sa VEL la

"Milhouse ran to Save Ella"

2009
$384–$476

❖ Serotonin-norepinephrine reuptake inhibitor (SNRI)
❖ Fibromyalgia medication
❖ 5-HT = NE

12.5
25
50
100
mg

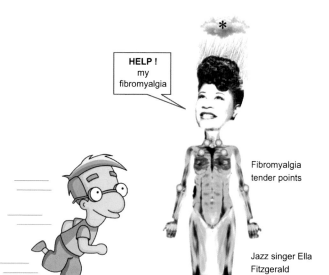

HELP !
my fibromyalgia

Fibromyalgia tender points

Jazz singer Ella Fitzgerald

Not approved for depression

FDA-approved for:
❖ Fibromyalgia

* Milnacipran (Savella) is the SNRI approved for fibromyalgia only, not for depression. It is properly referred to as an antidepressant and is approved for depression in some other countries. It has not shown robust antidepressant efficacy.

At the usual maintenance dose milnacipran is a "balanced" SNRI that enhances serotonin and norepinephrine activity by similar magnitude. At lower doses, e.g., 25 mg BID, noradrenergic effects are more pronounced than serotonergic effects.

Milnacipran is fairly well tolerated, with fewer gastrointestinal issues than SSRIs. Side effects that are more prominent with milnacipran (compared to SSRIs) include dizziness, sweating, and urinary hesitancy.

Levomilnacipran (Fetzima), the pure L-enantiomer of milnacipran, is FDA-approved for depression.

Of 236 single-drug exposures to milnacipran reported to Poison Control, there were 5 major serious outcomes but no deaths (Nelson & Spyker, 2017).

Dosing: Titrate to 50 mg BID using the starter pack shown below. Maximum dose is 200 mg (100 mg BID). Taper to discontinue to avoid unpleasant serotonin withdrawal symptoms.

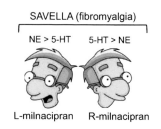

SAVELLA (fibromyalgia)

NE > 5-HT
L-milnacipran

5-HT > NE
R-milnacipran

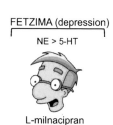

FETZIMA (depression)

NE > 5-HT
L-milnacipran

Savella is initiated by a titration that would be quite inconvenient without the "4 week convenience pack".

► 12.5 mg QD x 1 day,
► 12.5 mg BID x 2 days,
► 25 mg BID x 4 days,
► then 50 mg BID

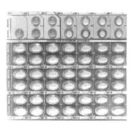

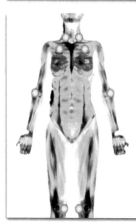

Medications for fibromyalgia

FDA-approved:
❖ Duloxetine (Cymbalta) – SNRI
❖ Milnacipran (Savella) – SNRI
❖ Pregabalin (Lyrica) – AED

Off-label:
❖ Venlafaxine (Effexor) – SNRI
❖ Gabapentin (Neurontin) – AED
❖ Amitriptyline (Elavil) – TCA
❖ Tramadol (Ultram) – weak opioid & SNRI

Dynamic interactions:
❖ Serotonergic
❖ Antiplatelet effect
❖ Hyponatremia
❖ Hypertension

Kinetic interactions:
❖ Milnacipran undergoes minimal CYP-related metabolism, with 55% of the dose excreted unchanged in urine. Kinetic interactions occur but are unlikely to be clinically relevant—"in a box".

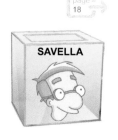

SAVELLA

page 18

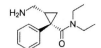

2013
$394–$484

Levomilnacipran (FETZIMA)
LEE voe mil NA si pran / fet ZEE ma

"Leave Milhouse with a Zima Fetish"

❖ Antidepressant
❖ Serotonin-norepinephrine reuptake inhibitor (SNRI)
❖ NE >> 5-HT

20
40
80
120
mg

FDA-approved for:
❖ Major depressive disorder

Used off-label for:
❖ Fibromyalgia
❖ Diabetic peripheral neuropathy
❖ Chronic musculoskeletal pain
❖ Vasomotor symptoms of menopause

Levomilnacipran (Fetzima), released in 2013, is the pure L-enantiomer of milnacipran (Savella). Fetzima will be expensive until the patent expires in 2031.

Compared to other SNRIs, levomilnacipran enhances norepinephrine >> serotonin, making it more stimulating. By contrast, milnacipran is a "balanced" SNRI that enhances serotonin and norepinephrine activity by similar magnitude at the usual maintenance dose.

Levomilnacipran causes no weight gain. The most relevant side effect is nausea, especially as treatment is initiated. This why the dose should be titrated. Dose dependent urinary retention (5%) and tachycardia and may occur. It increases heart rate by an average of 7 beats/minute, which is a noradrenergic effect.

Levomilnacipran was found effective in patients over age 60, a population that is generally resistant to antidepressants.

It reaches peak serum concentration about 7 hours after ingestion. Half-life is about 12 hours. Kinetic interactions are unlikely to be clinically significant.

Of 56 single-drug exposures to milnacipran reported to Poison Control, there were no deaths or major serious outcomes, although this is a small sample size (Nelson & Spyker, 2017).

Dosing: Start 20 mg QD x 2 days, then increase to 40 mg QD. This can be accomplished with the 28-day starter pack that contains #2 of 20 mg caps and #26 of 40 mg caps. FDA maximum is 120 mg QD if renal function is normal. Do not use if severe renal impairment. Do not exceed 80 mg/day in the presence of a strong 3A4 inHibitor (e.g., ketoconazole, clarithromycin, ritonavir). Taper gradually to discontinue.

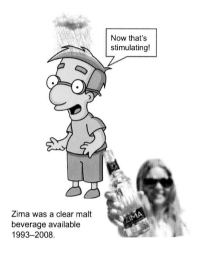

Now that's stimulating!

Zima was a clear malt beverage available 1993–2008.

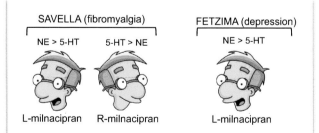

SAVELLA (fibromyalgia)

NE > 5-HT   5-HT > NE

L-milnacipran   R-milnacipran

FETZIMA (depression)

NE > 5-HT

L-milnacipran

Dynamic interactions:
❖ Serotonergic
❖ Antiplatelet effect
❖ Hyponatremia
❖ Hypertension

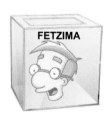

FETZIMA

page 18

Kinetic interactions:
❖ 85% is excreted in urine, 58% unchanged. Otherwise, it is primarily metabolized through 3A4/
❖ The package insert says not to exceed 80 mg/day in the presence of a strong 3A4 inHibitor (e.g., ketoconazole, clarithromycin, ritonavir). Otherwise, the max is 120 mg. The label for milnacipran (Savella) does not describe this interaction. As with Savella, we're putting Fetzima "in a box" to signify that kinetic interactions occur but are unlikely to be clinically significant.

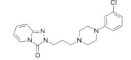

Trazodone (DESYREL)
TRA zo dohn / DES zi rel

"Trays o' bone / Dizzy reel"

❖ Antidepressant/sleep medication
❖ Serotonin antagonist and reuptake inhibitor (SARI)
 – 5-HT$_2$ antagonist
 – 5-HT$_{1A}$ agonist

50
100
150
300
mg

FDA-approved for:

❖ Major Depressive Disorder (MDD) —rarely used for this indication

Used off-label for:

❖ Insomnia (first-line)
❖ PTSD nightmares

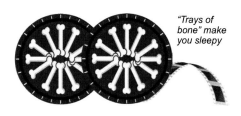

"Trays of bone" make you sleepy

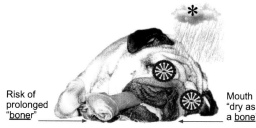

Risk of prolonged "boner"

Mouth "dry as a bone"

Trazodone (Desyrel) was the first non-tricyclic / non-MAOI antidepressant approved in the US, predating the SSRIs. Many psychiatrists consider trazodone their first-line sleep medication. It is the author's #1 most prescribed drug. It can be combined with any other medication. Low-dose Trazodone 50–75 mg can even be combined with an MAOI (Jacobsen, 1990). The author regards significantly prolonged QTc interval (over 490 msec or so) as the only contraindication.

Although it is approved as an antidepressant, trazodone is usually prescribed at low dose for insomnia, with no antidepressant benefit expected. It is seldom used as a stand-alone treatment for depression due to sedation and orthostatic hypotension if dosed at antidepressant strength. Trazodone is often prescribed as an adjunct to SSRIs. It may be helpful for reducing PTSD nightmares (Warner MD et al, 2001).

Trazodone induces and maintains sleep without causing tolerance. Its half-life of 3–6 hours is ideal for sleep without causing daytime drowsiness. The most common side effect is xerostomia—a mouth that's "dry as a bone". Most medications causing dry mouth do so as an anticholinergic effect. This is not the case with trazodone, which lacks anticholinergic effects.

It is a preferred sleep medication for those with obstructive sleep apnea (OSA) because it does not depress respiration. It does not cause weight gain or sexual side effects.

Many sedatives work by blocking H$_1$ histamine receptors. Trazodone is sedating due to a combination of moderate H$_1$ antihistamine effect plus antagonism of 5-HT$_{2A}$ and alpha-1 adrenergic receptors.

Priapism (painful prolonged erection) is a rare risk of Trazodone, and a medical emergency. Priapism is not considered a significant risk with any other psychotropic medication. Although the risk is low (1 in 6,000), think twice before prescribing trazodone to a man being discharged to jail, where prompt medical treatment for priapism might not be provided. Trazodone-induced priapism is likely attributable to antagonism of alpha-1 adrenoceptors, which interferes with the sympathetic control of penile detumescence.

Animal studies suggested trazodone could reduce the risk of dementia, but this does not appear to apply to humans (Brauer et al, 2019). At worst, trazodone does not contribute to dementia risk. Anticholinergic sleep medications like diphenhydramine (Benadryl) and doxylamine (Unisom) do increase risk of dementia.

The original trade name of trazodone was DESYREL, but no one calls it that because the generic name has such a nice ring to it. An extended-release version of trazodone branded as OLEPTRO (150, 300 mg) was available, but virtually no one prescribed it.

It is commonly misspelled as *trazadone*.

Dosing: Titrate slowly. The dose for insomnia is 25–200 mg, usually started at 50 mg, for routine or PRN use. For healthy adults, the author often prescribes 150 mg tablets with instructions to take ⅓ to 1 tab PRN which allows doses of 50, 75, 100, or 150 mg. QT prolongation may occur if the FDA max of 400 mg is exceeded. Antidepressant dosing is 300–600 mg, divided BID (as the label instructs) or taken all at HS which is better tolerated. 150 mg may be useful for depression for some patients.

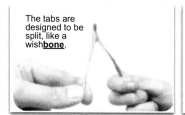

The tabs are designed to be split, like a wish**bone**.

All generic trazodone tabs are scored. The 150 mg and 300 mg generics are usually multi-scored:

50 mg generic

100 mg generic

Some 150 mg generics

300 mg generic

Dynamic interactions:

❖ Sedation/CNS depression
❖ QT prolongation (mild)

Kinetic interactions:

❖ We're depicting trazodone in a box because clinically significant kinetic interactions are unlikely, or at least not clearly defined. Trazodone is metabolized to m-chlorophenylpiperazine (mCPP) by 3A4. mCPP is then disposed of by 2D6. mCPP is a 5-HT agonist that can be associated with dysphoria, anxiety, and (rarely) hallucinations. mCPP only causes these effect when levels escalate quickly. Adding trazodone to a 2D6 inhibitor will rarely be an issue, especially if trazodone is started at a low dose for sleep. Adding a 2D6 inhibitor (e.g., fluoxetine, duloxetine, bupropion) to trazodone could cause transient anxiety/dysphoria by increasing mCPP abruptly. Note mCPP is also a metabolite of nefazodone, the other SARI antidepressant.
❖ Trazodone is an inducer of P-glycoprotein (P-gp), which pumps P-gp substrates out of the brain—"pumpers gonna pump"

page 18

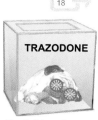

TRAZODONE

Kinetic interactions are rarely an issue

1994
$79–$173

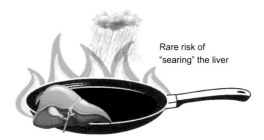

Nefazodone (SERZONE)
nef FAH zoe dohn / SARE zone
"Nefarious Sear zone"

❖ Antidepressant/sleep medication
❖ Serotonin antagonist and reuptake inhibitor (SARI)
  − 5-HT$_2$ antagonist
  − 5-HT$_{1A}$ agonist

50
100
150
<u>200</u>
250
mg

FDA-approved for:
❖ Major Depressive Disorder (MDD)

Rare risk of "searing" the liver

"The nefarious Trazodone"

Nefazodone (Serzone) is the second serotonin antagonist and reuptake inhibitor (SARI), developed as a <u>less sedating</u> derivative of <u>trazodone</u>. Nefazodone was released in 1994, and voluntarily withdrawn from market in 2004 by the original manufacturer due to decreasing sales related to **rare** <u>occurrences of severe liver damage</u>. The risk of severe liver damage is only 1 in every 250,000 to 300,000 patient-years.

Nefazodone is currently available, but rarely prescribed. It has a relatively mild side effect profile. Nefazodone has no anticholinergic activity, and only mildly antihistaminic. It does not cause priapism, which is a possible adverse event with trazodone. Nefazodone does not impair sexual functioning and may actually enhance it.

There are case reports of nefazodone causing <u>visual trailing</u>, which is a disturbance of motion perception where moving objects appear as a series of stroboscopic images. The illusion of trailing is common with LSD (via serotonergic mechanism), but is not associated with prescription psychotropic medications other than nefazodone.

Dosing: The target dose for depression is 200–300 mg divided BID, with max of 600 mg/day (300 mg BID); Start 100 mg BID; May increase by increments of 100–200 mg/day every week; Taper gradually to stop.

Dynamic interactions:
❖ Serotonergic

Kinetic interactions:
❖ Nefazodone is a potent 3A4 inhibitor, raising levels of some 3A4 substrates 5-fold. Trazodone does not do this.
❖ Nefazodone is a competitive inhibitor of 3A4, i.e., nefazodone is itself a 3A4 substrate.
❖ Nefazodone is metabolized to m-<u>c</u>hloro<u>p</u>henyl<u>p</u>iperazine (mCPP). Refer to the trazodone monograph for the possible significance of mCPP.

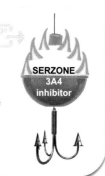

page 16

SERZONE
3A4 inhibitor

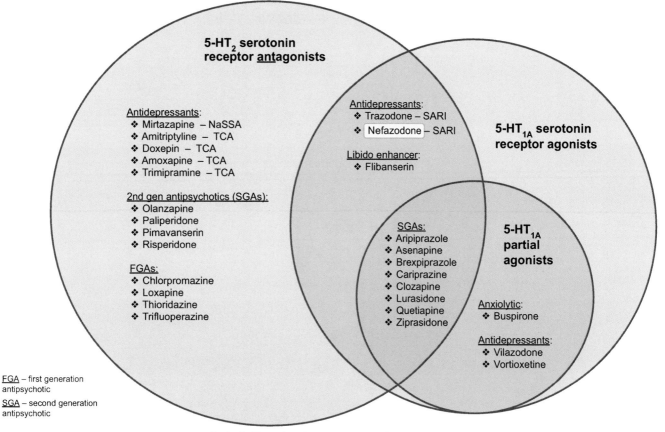

5-HT$_2$ serotonin receptor <u>ant</u>agonists

Antidepressants:
❖ Mirtazapine – NaSSA
❖ Amitriptyline – TCA
❖ Doxepin – TCA
❖ Amoxapine – TCA
❖ Trimipramine – TCA

2nd gen antipsychotics (SGAs):
❖ Olanzapine
❖ Paliperidone
❖ Pimavanserin
❖ Risperidone

FGAs:
❖ Chlorpromazine
❖ Loxapine
❖ Thioridazine
❖ Trifluoperazine

Antidepressants:
❖ Trazodone – SARI
❖ Nefazodone – SARI

Libido enhancer:
❖ Flibanserin

5-HT$_{1A}$ serotonin receptor agonists

SGAs:
❖ Aripiprazole
❖ Asenapine
❖ Brexpiprazole
❖ Cariprazine
❖ Clozapine
❖ Lurasidone
❖ Quetiapine
❖ Ziprasidone

5-HT$_{1A}$ partial agonists

Anxiolytic:
❖ Buspirone

Antidepressants:
❖ Vilazodone
❖ Vortioxetine

<u>F</u>GA – first generation antipsychotic

<u>S</u>GA – second generation antipsychotic

#128
1996
$9–$52

Mirtazapine (REMERON)

mir TAZ ah peen / rim er ON

"Mr Taz zapping (R.E.M.-a'roni)"

❖ Noradrenergic and Specific
   Serotonergic Antidepressant
   (NaSSA)
   – Alpha-2 antagonist
   – 5-HT$_2$ antagonist
   – 5-HT$_3$ antagonist

7.5
15
30
45
mg

FDA-approved for:

❖ Major depressive disorder

Used off-label for:

❖ SSRI-induced sexual dysfunction
❖ Appetite stimulation
❖ Akathisia

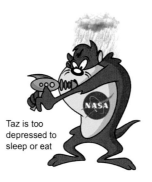

Taz is too
depressed to
sleep or eat

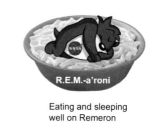

Eating and sleeping
well on Remeron

Mirtazapine (Remeron) is a noradrenergic and specific serotonergic (5-HT) antidepressant (NaSSA) with a relatively high response rate and low dropout rate (Cipriani et al, 2018). It is an antagonist at norepinephrine (alpha-2), 5-HT$_2$, and 5-HT$_3$ receptors. Mirtazapine is a suitable first-line antidepressant option for an underweight patient who can't sleep. Mirtazapine has antiemetic properties thanks to 5-HT$_3$ antagonism, which is the principal mechanism of action of ondansetron (Zofran).

Remeron is a potent antihistamine, leading to sedation and appetite stimulation. About half of patients gain significant weight. However, at higher doses, its noradrenergic characteristics outshine its antihistamine effects. Hence, at high doses mirtazepine can be *less* sedating and cause *less* appetite stimulation. This is a unusual property among psychotropics, also noted with the TCA doxepin (Sinequan).

Mirtazapine may work a bit faster than other antidepressants. The patient will "remember" the prescriber fondly for making them feel better quickly with Remeron, then not so fondly for making them fat. Consider using Remeron for an acute depressive episode, then changing to another antidepressant (or increasing the dose of mirtazapine) if the patient starts gaining weight.

"California Rocket Fuel" is a combination of mirtazapine with the SNRI venlafaxine (Effexor). This combo was previously felt to be exceptionally effective for depression due to complementary mechanisms of action. Unfortunately, mirtazapine augmentation was recently found to be no better than placebo for individuals who had failed antidepressant monotherapy (Navarro et al, 2019).

Mirtazapine is a third-line treatment for akathisia (behind propranolol and clonazepam) at 15 mg. At higher doses mirtazapine may exacerbate akathisia. Other side effects of mirtazapine include dry mouth and constipation. There is a risk of neutropenia, although rare.

Remeron does not inhibit sexual functioning, and can actually be used as an adjunct to reverse SSRI-induced sexual dysfunction.

Dosing: Start 15 mg HS; FDA maximum is 45 mg, but 60 mg is safe and may be more effective for depression. Note that mirtazapine causes less somnolence and less weight gain at higher doses. For treatment of akathisia, do not exceed 15 mg.

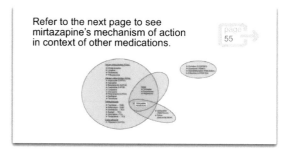

Refer to the next page to see mirtazapine's mechanism of action in context of other medications.

page 55

Dynamic interactions:

❖ Sedation/CNS depression (strong)
❖ QT prolongation (mild)
❖ Serotonergic effects (weak)
❖ Alpha-2 adrenoceptor antagonist
   – Do not add **mirtazapine** to alpha-2 agonists such **clonidine** (Catapres) or **guanfacine** (Tenex) because mirtazapine will block the effect of the alpha-2 agonist, potentially leading to hypertensive rebound. Do not add an alpha-2 agonist to Remeron, because the alpha-2 agonist may be ineffective.

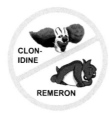

CLON-
IDINE

REMERON

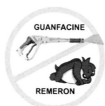

GUANFACINE

REMERON

Kinetic interactions:

❖ Mirtazapine is metabolized by several CYP enzymes (1A2,2D6, 3A4). Kinetic interactions occur but are unlikely to be clinically significant.

page 18

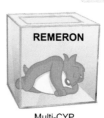

REMERON

Multi-CYP

Cafer's Psychopharmacology | cafermed.com

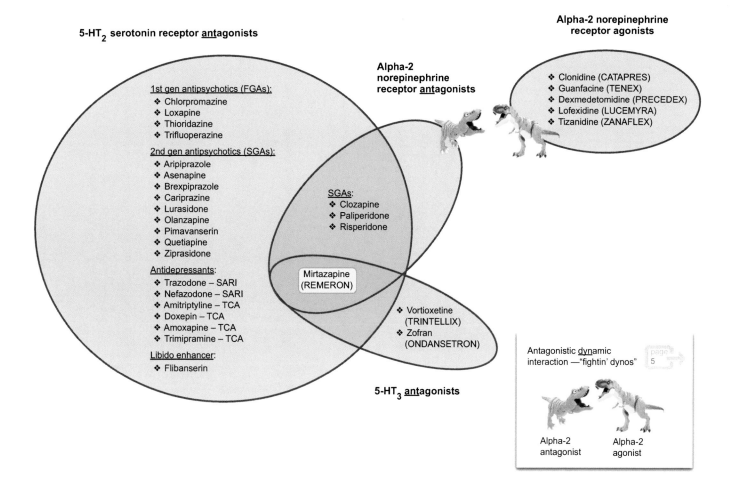

5-HT$_2$ serotonin receptor <u>ant</u>agonists

1st gen antipsychotics (FGAs):
- Chlorpromazine
- Loxapine
- Thioridazine
- Trifluoperazine

2nd gen antipsychotics (SGAs):
- Aripiprazole
- Asenapine
- Brexpiprazole
- Cariprazine
- Lurasidone
- Olanzapine
- Pimavanserin
- Quetiapine
- Ziprasidone

Antidepressants:
- Trazodone – SARI
- Nefazodone – SARI
- Amitriptyline – TCA
- Doxepin – TCA
- Amoxapine – TCA
- Trimipramine – TCA

Libido enhancer:
- Flibanserin

Alpha-2 norepinephrine receptor <u>ant</u>agonists

SGAs:
- Clozapine
- Paliperidone
- Risperidone

Mirtazapine (REMERON)

- Vortioxetine (TRINTELLIX)
- Zofran (ONDANSETRON)

5-HT$_3$ <u>ant</u>agonists

Alpha-2 norepinephrine receptor agonists
- Clonidine (CATAPRES)
- Guanfacine (TENEX)
- Dexmedetomidine (PRECEDEX)
- Lofexidine (LUCEMYRA)
- Tizanidine (ZANAFLEX)

Antagonistic <u>dyn</u>amic interaction —"fightin' dynos"

Alpha-2 antagonist   Alpha-2 agonist

California Rocket Fuel

SNRI + NaSSA

Venlafaxine (EFFEXOR) + Mirtazapine (REMERON)

- Antidepressant combination

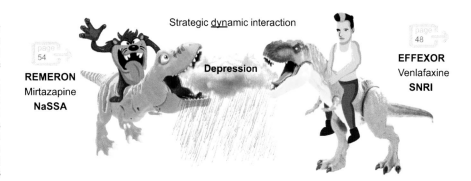

Strategic <u>dyn</u>amic interaction

REMERON Mirtazapine **NaSSA**   Depression   **EFFEXOR** Venlafaxine **SNRI**

"California Rocket Fuel", popularized by psychiatrist Stephen Stahl, is a combination of venlafaxine (SNRI) and mirtazapine (noradrenergic and specific serotonergic antidepressant, NaSSA). This combination boosts serotonin and norepinephrine neurotransmission in multiple ways. The STAR-D study found this combination to be at least as effective as the MAOI tranylcypromine (Parnate). In a series of 32 patients with refractory depression, 44% responded at four weeks and 50% at eight weeks (Hannan et al, 2007). The combination was generally well tolerated, although 12% of patients reported moderate to severe weight gain and, 12% reported at least moderate sedation.

Unfortunately, larger studies were <u>disappointing</u>. For 112 patients who failed to respond to venlafaxine, remission rate was 39% when mirtazapine was added, compared to 72% when venlafaxine was changed to the TCA imipramine (Navarro et al, 2019).

This "heroic" treatment should be prescribed with caution due to risk of serotonin syndrome. California Rocket Fuel should be reserved for treatment of refractory <u>unipolar</u> depression. The combo should not be given to patients with a personal or family history of bipolar disorder due to risk of precipitating mania.

A similar combination of the SNRI <u>duloxetine</u> (Cymbalta) with mirtazapine has been referred to as "<u>Limerick Rocket Fuel</u>".

Dosing: In a case series, most patients who responded were titrated to relatively high doses of both medications —venlafaxine ER at least 225 mg/day and mirtazapine 30–45 mg HS.

Bottom line: There appears to be <u>nothing magical</u> about this combination. This combination is an example of two antidepressants with mechanisms that are synergistic on paper but disappointing in practice. See page 23 for proven options for treatment-resistant depression.

#260
2013
$357–$462

Vortioxetine (TRINTELLIX)
vor tye OX e teen / trin TELL ix

"Trent's Vortex"

❖ Multimodal antidepressant
❖ Serotonin modulator and stimulator (SMS)
  - 5-HT reuptake inhibitor
  - 5-HT$_{1A}$ partial agonist
  - 5-HT$_3$ antagonist

5
10
20
mg

FDA-approved for:
❖ Major depressive disorder

Used off-label for:
❖ OCD

"Serotonergic vortex"—Vortioxetine (Trintellix) is a "serotonin modulator and stimulator" (SMS) approved in 2013 for treatment of depression. The original trade name was BRINTELLIX, suggestive of *"Bring Intelligence"*. In 2016 the trade name was changed to Trintellix to avoid confusion with antiplatelet drug BRILINTA (ticagrelor).

Although expensive, Trinetellix is a reasonable first-line option for depression if cognitive deficits are prominent. Cognitive dysfunction characteristic of profound depression can be referred to as pseudodementia. Trintellix's marketing slogan is *"fight the fog of depression"*, which refers to its ability to improve pseudodementia. This is useful because, on average, depression impairs cognition similarly to 24 hours of sleep deprivation (Mahableshwarkar et al, 2016). Vortioxetine improves cognition, although the effect is modest, roughly equivalent to 50 mg of caffeine (Jaeger et al, 2018).

Side effects: Vortioxetine is relatively well-tolerated. At the suggested maintenance dose of 20 mg, incidence of sexual dysfunction is 44%. At 10 mg vortioxetine has fewer sexual side effects than SSRIs. Vortioxetine is more likely to cause constipation than diarrhea. Headache and dizziness have been reported. It does not cause weight gain or prolong QT interval. Vortioxetine appears to be among the safest psychotropic medications in overdose, with no known deaths, although sample size is small. Due to long half-life of 3 days, it does not cause discontinuation symptoms with missed doses.

About 30% of patients experience nausea, as could be expected from a "vortex" of serotonergic mechanisms. Nausea due to antidepressants (including vortioxetine) typically resolves after a couple of weeks. Nausea with vortioxetine is tempered by 5-HT$_3$ antagonism. Other drugs that block 5-HT$_3$ include the antiemetic ondansetron (Zofran) and the NaSSA antidepressant mirtazapine (Remeron). Ginger also relieves nausea via the same mechanism.

Dosing: The starting dose is 10 mg. The suggested maintenance dose for MDD is 20 mg, but staying at 10 mg may be adequate, with fewer side effects.

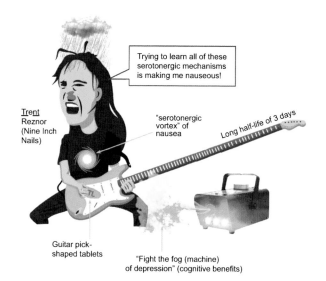

Trent Reznor (Nine Inch Nails)

Trying to learn all of these serotonergic mechanisms is making me nauseous!

"serotonergic vortex" of nausea

Long half-life of 3 days

Guitar pick-shaped tablets

"Fight the fog (machine) of depression" (cognitive benefits)

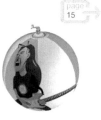

Dynamic interactions:
❖ Serotonergic effects (strong)
❖ Antiplatelet effects
❖ Hyponatremia

Kinetic interactions:
❖ 2D6 substrate
❖ 2D6 poor metabolizers should not exceed 10 mg.
❖ Vortioxetine levels are doubled by bupropion (Wellbutrin), which is a strong 2D6 inHibitor.

2D6 substrate

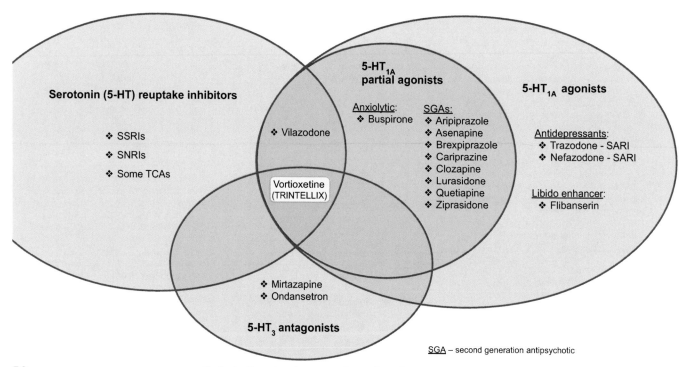

Serotonin (5-HT) reuptake inhibitors

❖ SSRIs
❖ SNRIs
❖ Some TCAs

❖ Vilazodone

5-HT$_{1A}$ partial agonists

Anxiolytic:
❖ Buspirone

SGAs:
❖ Aripiprazole
❖ Asenapine
❖ Brexpiprazole
❖ Cariprazine
❖ Clozapine
❖ Lurasidone
❖ Quetiapine
❖ Ziprasidone

5-HT$_{1A}$ agonists

Antidepressants:
❖ Trazodone - SARI
❖ Nefazodone - SARI

Libido enhancer:
❖ Flibanserin

Vortioxetine (TRINTELLIX)

❖ Mirtazapine
❖ Ondansetron

5-HT$_3$ antagonists

SGA – second generation antipsychotic

Cafer's Psychopharmacology | cafermed.com

Vilazodone (VIIBRYD)

vil AZ o dohn / VY brid

"(what that) Vile lazer done (to that) Virile hybrid"

❖ Antidepressant
❖ Serotonin Modulator and Stimulator (SMS)
- 5-HT reuptake inhibitor (SRI)
- 5-HT$_{1A}$ partial agonist

10
20
40
mg

FDA-approved for:
❖ Major depressive disorder

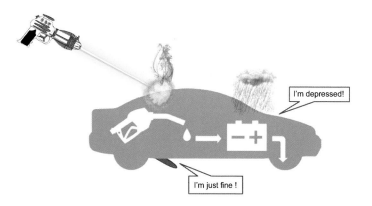

I'm depressed!

I'm just fine !

Vilazodone (Viibryd) is an atypical antidepressant released in 2011. It was described as the first serotonin partial agonist/reuptake inhibitor (SPARI). Alternately, it can be grouped with vortioxetine (Trintellix, 2013) as a serotonin modulator and stimulator (SMS). Vilazodone is less complicated than vortioxetine in terms of mechanism of action.

"Virile" Viibryd was marketed as having fewer sexual side effects than SSRIs, though it does cause slightly more sexual dysfunction than placebo.

Viibryd's mechanism is a "Hybrid" an SSRI and a 5-HT$_{1A}$ partial agonist. In other words, vilazodone combines the pharmacologic actions of an SSRI and the anxiolytic buspirone (Buspar). SSRIs are famously detrimental to sexual functioning. Buspirone improves sexually functioning. To concoct a "Poor Man's Viibryd", prescribe buspirone with the purest SSRI, escitalopram (Lexapro).

Until it goes generic, Viibryd is $300/month, and is unproven to be superior to an SSRI for treatment of depression.

Vilazodone needs to be taken with food for adequate absorption. Only 50% of the dose is absorbed on an empty stomach.

At 40 mg/day, the most common adverse effects are diarrhea (28% vs 9% placebo), nausea (23% vs 5% placebo), and insomnia (6% vs 2% placebo).

Dosing: Target dose is 20–40 mg QD with food. Must titrate with 10 mg QD for the first week, as shown below. The 30-day starter pack contains 10 mg tab x 7 and 20 mg tab x 23. To discontinue, taper off over about a week.

To avoid side effects, vilazodone needs to be titrated.

10   10 mg QD for days 1–7

20   20 mg QD day 8 onward

40   40 mg QD as early as day 15 onward (versus staying at 20 mg)

The 3 psychotropic medications that must be taken **with food** for adequate absorption—the *DONE-nuts*.

❖ Vilazo<u>done</u> (VIIBRYD) - antidepressant
❖ Ziprasi<u>done</u> (GEODON) - antipsychotic
❖ Lurasi<u>done</u> (LATUDA) - antipsychotic

Without food, absorption is only 50%.

"Poor Man's Viibryd"

An approximation of vilazodone's mechanism of action can be achieved by co-prescribing escitalopram and buspirone.

Escitalopram (Lexapro)
SSRI
$10
sexual dysfunction

Buspirone (Buspar)
5-HT$_{1A}$ partial agonist
$10
sexual enhancement

"Bus spear"

Vilazodone (Viibryd)
SRI + 5-HT$_{1A}$ partial agonist
$300
minimal sexual dysfunction

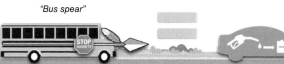

Vilazodone causes slightly more sexual dysfunction than placebo.

Here are some medications that can actually improve sexual functioning:

❖ Trazodone (Desyrel)
❖ Nefazodone (Serzone)
❖ Mirtazapine (Remeron)
❖ Bupropion (Wellbutrin)
❖ Buspirone (BuSpar) - anxiolytic

Dynamic interactions:
❖ Serotonergic effects (strong)
❖ Antiplatelet effects
❖ Hyponatremia

Kinetic interactions:
❖ 3A4 substrate (major)

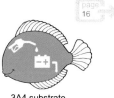

3A4 substrate

page 16

Serotonin Discontinuation Syndrome
"withdrawal" if an antidepressant is stopped abruptly

Serotonergic antidepressants are nonaddictive, but "withdrawal" symptoms may occur upon discontinuation, especially if the course of treatment has been > 2 months. Serotonin discontinuation syndrome includes flu-like symptoms, irritability, and unusual sensations described as "brain zaps". Serotonin withdrawal is unpleasant but not physically dangerous. It is more likely with serotonergics of short half-life, such as paroxetine (Paxil), venlafaxine (Effexor), and fluvoxamine (Luvox). Discontinuation syndrome is problematic even with extended-release Effexor XR. These unpleasant side effects can be avoided if the antidepressant is tapered to discontinue. Some patients may require a long-tail taper over several months to avoid serotonin withdrawal symptoms.

Venlafaxine (Effexor)

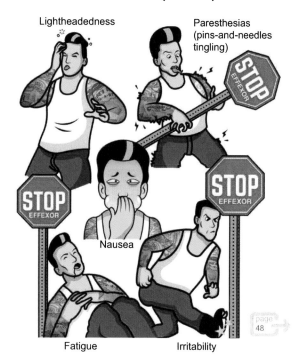

Paroxetine (Paxil)

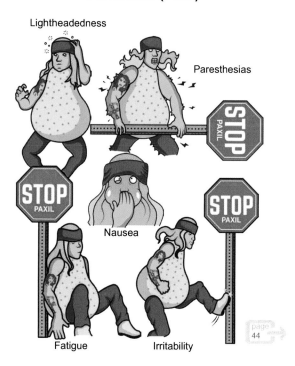

Fluvoxamine (Luvox)

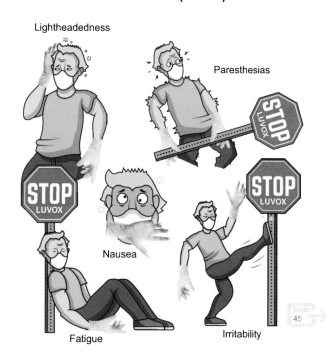

Linear tapering

Psychiatrists have traditionally tapered off antidepressants linearly, for instance decreasing from 40 mg to 30 mg x 1 week, then 20 mg x 1 week, then 10 mg x 1 week. Linear tapers are not ideal, often providing minimal benefit over abrupt discontinuation for avoiding serotonin withdrawal symptoms.

Hyperbolic tapering

 Horowitz & Taylor in *The Lancet Psychiatry* (June 2019) explain a more effective approach, referred to as the hyperbolic taper (as traditionally used to get off of benzodiazepines). Hyperbolic tapering involves a quick decrease to the usual starting dose, then a long-tail taper over a period of months, getting down to tiny doses well below the therapeutic range.

To get low-enough doses you need to use a compounding pharmacy, liquid formulations, or chop tablets into tiny fragments. Capsules are not ideal, but a patient who understands the concept could open them, discard an inexact fraction of the medication and reassemble.

Among SSRIs, liquid formulations are available for citalopram, escitalopram, fluoxetine, and sertraline (but not for fluvoxamine or paroxetine).

For the nitty gritty on parabolic tapering, Refer to my favorite newsletter, *The Carlat Psychiatry Report* (Drs Sazima & Aiken, Jun/Jul 2019).

Catecholamines

Neurotransmitter	Abbrev	Normal activity	Low activity	High activity	Comments
Norepinephrine	NE	Energy, Motivation, Ability to focus and respond to stress	Fatigue Inattention Sexual dysfunction	Insomnia Anxiety Loss of appetite Hypertension Seizure	NE is also known as noradrenaline. Stimulants increase noradrenergic (NE) activity.
Dopamine	DA	Ability to experience pleasure and strong emotions	Anhedonia, Inattention, Sexual dysfunction, Parkinsonism, Akathisia, Dystonia, Neuroleptic malignant syndrome (NMS), Restless legs syndrome	Mania, Euphoria, Agitation, Anger, Aggression, Chemical "high", Paranoia, Auditory hallucinations, Hypersexuality, Insomnia, Compulsive behaviors	Think pleasure, passion, paranoia. Drugs of abuse, colloquially known as "dope", cause euphoria by spiking DA in the nucleus accumbens.

Norepinephrine reuptake inhibitors (NRIs)

NRIs increase the availability of norepinephrine (NE) in the extracellular space. NE is energizing and may contribute to hypertension.

NRI	Main use	Comments
Atomoxetine (STRATTERA)	ADHD	Non-controlled substance; Less effective for ADHD than Schedule II stimulants; Rare hepatotoxicity

Some tricyclic antidepressants (TCAs) are NRIs by mechanism. While other TCAs are anxiety-reducing, these are drive-enhancing. Since TCAs are non-selective, their stimulating effects are tempered by antihistaminic effects. These noradrenergic TCAs *could* be co-prescribed with a monoamine oxidase inhibitor (MAOI) without causing serotonin syndrome, but expect the pharmacist to flip out. Taking serotonergic TCAs (amitriptyline, imipramine, clomipramine) with an MAOI could be catastrophic.

Tricyclic (TCA)	Main use	Comments
Nortriptyline (PAMELOR)	Depression Migraine prevention	The major active metabolite of amitriptyline. While amitriptyline is sedating, nortriptyline (like all medications on this page) is stimulating. It is safer and better tolerated than most TCAs.
Desipramine (NORPRAMIN)	Depression	Exceptionally fatal in overdose.
Maprotiline (LUDIOMIL)	Depression	Rarely prescribed. Tetracyclic structure. Most likely to induce seizures among available antidepressants.

Dopamine (or dopamine/norepinephrine) reuptake inhibitors

Norepinephrine-dopamine reuptake inhibitors (NDRIs) block reuptake of NE > DA

NDRI	Main use	Comments
Bupropion (WELLBUTRIN)	Depression Smoking cessation	Non-controlled; In addition to inhibiting reuptake of NE and DA, bupropion is a NE and DA releaser (NE > DA); Used off-label for ADHD and for SSRI associated sexual dysfunction.
Solriamfetol (SUNOSI)	Daytime sleepiness	Schedule IV controlled

Dopamine-norepinephrine reuptake inhibitors (DNRIs) block reuptake of DA > NE

DNRI	Main use	Comments
Methylphenidate (RITALIN)	ADHD	Schedule II controlled
Amphetamine (ADDERALL)	ADHD	Schedule II controlled; Also DA and NE release (DA > NE)
Lisdexamfetamine (VYVANSE)	ADHD Binge-eating disorder	Schedule II controlled; Also DA and NE release (DA > NE); Long-acting amphetamine less likely to be abused because of delayed onset of action. It is a prodrug converted to dextroamphetamine in red blood cells.
Dasotraline (trade name to be announced)	Binge-eating disorder	FDA-accepted 2019 for binge-eating disorder; It failed approval for ADHD

Dopamine reuptake inhibitors (DRIs) block reuptake of DA but not NE

DRI	Main use	Comments
Modafinil (PROVIGIL)	Daytime sleepiness	Schedule IV controlled; Binds dopamine transporter weakly
Armodafinil (NUVIGIL)	Daytime sleepiness	Schedule IV controlled; R-enantiomer of modafinil

Atomoxetine (STRATTERA)
at om OX e tine / stra TARE uh

"Atomic Stratosphere"

❖ ADHD medication
❖ Norepinephrine reuptake inhibitor (NRI)
❖ Non-controlled

10 mg
18
25
40
60
80
100

Not an antidepressant

FDA-approved for:
❖ Attention-deficit/ hyperactivity disorder (ADHD) ≥ 6 years old

Used off-label for:
❖ Cataplexy
❖ Dyslexia

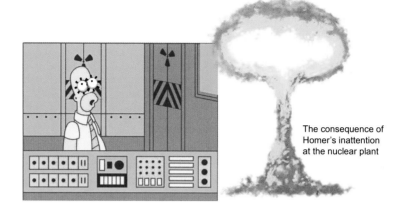

The consequence of Homer's inattention at the nuclear plant

Strattera straightens out your attention. Atomoxetine (Strattera) is a norepinephrine reuptake inhibitor (NRI) with the sole FDA-approved indication of ADHD. Although atomoxetine is not properly referred to as an antidepressant, it resides in the antidepressant chapter because its mechanism is similar to some antidepressants used off-label for ADHD including bupropion (Wellbutrin) and TCAs such as desipramine, nortriptyline, and protriptyline.

Although it has stimulating properties, atomoxetine is referred to as a "non-stimulant" to contrast it with the Schedule II ADHD stimulants (amphetamine, methylphenidate). Atomoxetine is not a controlled substance.

By inhibiting the norepinephrine transporter (NET), atomoxetine indirectly increases dopamine (DA) transmission in the prefrontal cortex (which is underactive with ADHD) without increasing DA in the nucleus accumbens (reward center). Therefore atomoxetine has no abuse potential because it does not increase DA in the nucleus accumbens.

When used to augment an SSRI, atomoxetine has the potential to improve anxiety and depression. Atomoxetine appears to improve reading skills in children with dyslexia (Shaywitz et al, 2017).

Atomoxetine poses a risk of suicidality in children/adolescents with ADHD, especially during the first months of treatment. Average risk of suicidal thoughts was 0.4% with atomoxetine vs 0% with placebo, but no suicides were reported. All antidepressants have a similar warning about suicide, which is another reason atomoxetine resides in this chapter. Other treatments for ADHD (Adderall, Ritalin, Tenex, Intuniv, etc) do not have this boxed warning.

Advantages of Strattera over Schedule II stimulants for treatment of ADHD:

► not a controlled substance
► no abuse potential
► does not worsen tics
► less likely to cause insomnia

Disadvantages:

► Less effective than stimulants—40% of patients are left with residual ADHD symptoms.
► Initial therapeutic effects are not seen until 2–4 weeks (whereas Schedule II stimulants work immediately).
► Rare risk of serious hepatic injury

Side effects of atomoxetine include headache, abdominal pain, and nausea. It may increase BP and heart rate.

If atomoxetine is stopped abruptly, withdrawal or other issues are not expected.

A similar "non-stimulant" option for off-label treatment of ADHD is the stimulating antidepressant bupropion (Wellbutrin), which has fewer risks and side effects than Strattera.

Adult dosing: For ADHD the target dose is 80 mg/day, either q AM or divided BID; Start 40 mg AM for at least 3 days, then may increase to maximum dose of 100 mg/day after 2–4 weeks; Use a lower dose with individuals who are known CYP2D6 poor metabolizers. When stopping, a gradual taper is considered unnecessary.

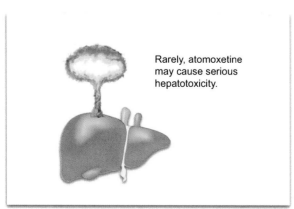

Rarely, atomoxetine may cause serious hepatotoxicity.

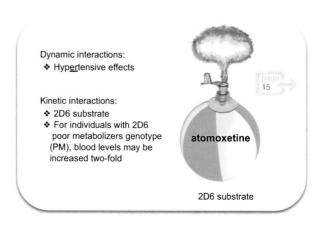

Dynamic interactions:
❖ Hypertensive effects

Kinetic interactions:
❖ 2D6 substrate
❖ For individuals with 2D6 poor metabolizers genotype (PM), blood levels may be increased two-fold

atomoxetine

2D6 substrate

page 15

#28
1985
XL $12–$109 (#30)
SR $9–$76 (#60)

Bupropion (WELLBUTRIN)
bu PRO pi on / wel BYU trin
"Boop ropin' Well booty"

❖ Antidepressant
❖ Norepinephrine-
   dopamine reuptake
   inhibitor (NDRI)
❖ Non-controlled

SR:
100
150
200
mg

XL:
150
300
mg

FDA-approved for:

❖ Major depressive disorder
❖ Seasonal affective disorder
❖ Smoking cessation
   (Zyban brand)

Used off-label for:

❖ ADHD
❖ Appetite suppression/
   weight loss
❖ SSRI-associated sexual
   dysfunction

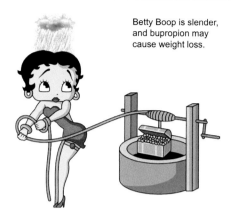

Betty Boop is slender,
and bupropion may
cause weight loss.

"Wellbutrin helps your mood get well". Bupropion (Wellbutrin), the #28 most prescribed overall medication, is a stimulating antidepressant that enhances norepinephrine and dopamine activity. Unlike most other modern antidepressants, it does not enhance serotonin activity. It is used for smoking cessation because it is stimulating like nicotine. These stimulating properties also make it useful for ADHD. Bupropion has demonstrated cognitive benefits. Clinicians tend to avoid prescribing it to individuals with anxiety disorders, but despite its stimulating properties, bupropion does not appear to exacerbate anxiety (Wiseman, 2012).

The serotonergic antidepressants cause sexual dysfunction. Bupropion is not serotonergic and actually improves sexual functioning. It is used as an add-on to SSRIs to ameliorate sexual problems (off-label).

Bupropion is contraindicated in patients with a current or prior diagnosis of bulimia or anorexia because of a higher reported incidence of seizures in such patients taking Wellbutrin.

Wellbutrin suppresses appetite and may cause modest weight loss. As with other stimulant-type medications, bupropion decreases appetite via adrenergic and dopaminergic receptors in the hypothalamus. The incidence of weight loss greater than 5 pounds is about 28%. CONTRAVE is a fixed-dose combination of bupropion with the opioid antagonist naltrexone, approved for long term treatment of obesity.

If taken by individuals with bipolar disorder, bupropion appears less likely to induce mania compared to serotonergic antidepressants.

Bupropion's chemical structure is similar to synthetic "bath salt" drugs. Wellbutrin is not a controlled substance and is not generally considered a drug of abuse. It increases dopamine levels in the prefrontal cortex (underactive in ADHD) but not in the nucleus accumbens (reward center), at least not at standard doses. However, bupropion is avoided by many prescribers in correctional facilities because inmates have collected tabs to crush and snort as "poor man's cocaine".

Bupropion, an NDRI, is a much weaker inhibitor of DA and NE reuptake than the Schedule II controlled stimulants approved for ADHD like methylphenidate (Ritalin) and amphetamine (Adderall). Ritalin and Adderall are referred to as DNRIs because their dopaminergic effect is stronger than their noradrenergic effect. Solriamfetol (Sunosi), approved for excessive daytime sleepiness (due to narcolepsy or sleep apnea) is a Schedule IV NDRI.

Bupropion has anti-inflammatory properties as a tumor necrosis factor (TNF) inhibitor. For treatment-resistant depression, adding bupropion to an SSRI is effective for patients who are overweight or have high C-reactive protein (CRP), a marker of inflammation (Jha MK, 2017). Otherwise, adding bupropion to an SSRI appears to be of no benefit for treatment-resistant depressant.

Risk of overdose mortality with bupropion is higher than with most other modern antidepressants. Of 51,118 single-drug exposures to bupropion reported to Poison Control, there were 3,239 major serious outcomes and 47 deaths (Nelson & Spyker, 2017).

Dosing:

Formulation	Dosing	Starting dose	Usual target dose	Max	To minimize seizure risk:
Wellbutrin XL (bupropion ER)	QD	150 mg AM	300 mg AM	450 mg AM	XL (ER) is the preferred formulation because seizure risk is minimal.
Wellbutrin SR	BID	100 mg BID	150 mg BID	400 mg/day = 200 mg BID	Separate doses by at least 8 hours.
Wellbutrin IR	TID	75 mg TID	100 mg TID	450 mg/day = 150 mg TID	Not recommended due to seizure risk, except for gastric bypass patients. Separate doses by at least 6 hours.

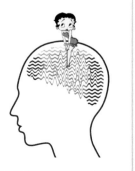

Bupropion may cause **seizures** at high doses or with the immediate-release formulation. Convulsant effect of standard doses of extended-release bupropion is minimal (Alper et al, 2007).

The maximum dose of Wellbutrin XL is 450 mg, taken once daily in the morning. This is typically accomplished with a 300 mg plus 150 mg tablet, or by three 150's. An expensive 450 mg tablet branded as FORFIVO exists. It is only mentioned for the cute name (4-5-0), and to aid in remembering the maximum dose of Wellbutrin XL.

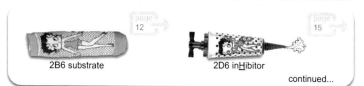

2B6 substrate

2D6 inHibitor

page 12

page 15

continued...

page 12
page 15

Bupropion (Wellbutrin)

Dynamic interactions:
- ❖ CNS stimulation
- ❖ Hy<u>per</u>tensive effects
- ❖ Lowers seizure threshold

Kinetic interactions:
- ❖ 2B6 in<u>H</u>ibitor (strong)
- ❖ 2B6 substrate
- ❖ Active metabolite hydroxy-bupropion is a 2D6 substrate (see below)

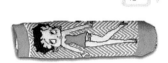

2B6 substrate

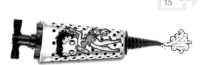

2D6 in<u>H</u>ibitor (strong)

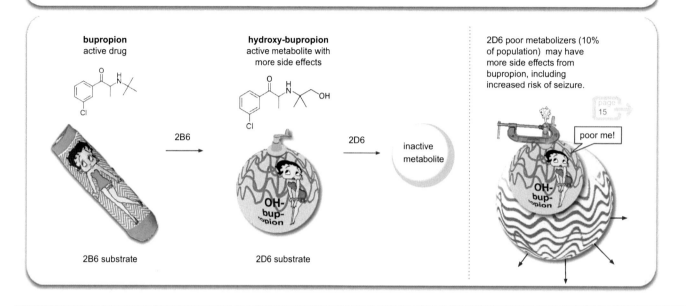

bupropion
active drug

hydroxy-bupropion
active metabolite with more side effects

2B6

2D6

inactive metabolite

2D6 poor metabolizers (10% of population) may have more side effects from bupropion, including increased risk of seizure.

page 15

poor me!

2B6 substrate

2D6 substrate

2019
$657–$714

Solriamfetol (SUNOSI)

SOL ri AM fe tol / su NO see

"Sun nosey with Solar feet"

- ❖ Norepinephrine-dopamine reuptake inhibitor (NDRI)
- ❖ Schedule IV

75
<u>150</u>
mg

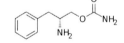

Not an antidepressant

FDA-approved for:
- ❖ Excessive daytime sleepiness due to:
  - Narcolepsy
  - Obstructive sleep apnea (OSA)

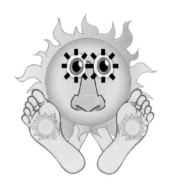

Solriamfetol (Sunosi) is a new <u>wakefulness promoting</u> medication that lasts for <u>9 hours</u>. It is stimulating but not considered a "stimulant". It is a norepinephrine and weak dopamine reuptake inhibitor. Sunosi could be conceptualized as an atypical antidepressant with a mechanism similar bupropion (Wellbutrin). However, solriamfetol is <u>not approved for depression</u>, and clinical trials did <u>not include psychiatric patients</u>. About 1 in 25 subjects treated for narcolepsy/sleep apnea had psychiatric side effects such as irritability and anxiety.

Solriamfetol is a <u>Schedule IV controlled</u> substance. By comparison, bupropion is non-controlled but does have potential for abuse at high doses.

Subjects who abused drugs reported "drug liking" similar to the appetite-suppressing stimulant phentermine (Adipex) when solriamfetol was taken at supratherapeutic dose. Phentermine is also Schedule IV.

Other effects include nausea and <u>appetite suppression</u>. It may increase blood pressure and heart rate.

An advantage over bupropion is that solriamfetol is free from significant kinetic drug/drug interactions.

The two other wakefulness promoters approved for narcolepsy/sleep apnea are modafinil (Provigil) and armodafinil (Nuvigil), which are also Schedule IV. For context, methylphenidate (Ritalin) and amphetamine (Adderall) are more strictly regulated as Schedule II controlled substances, and are referred to as stimulants.

Dosing: Start 75 mg q AM. Dose may be increased to 150 mg after 3 days based on efficacy and tolerability. Maximum dose is 150 mg/day.

page 18

Dynamic interactions:
- ❖ Dopaminergic
- ❖ Hy<u>per</u>tensive

Kinetic interactions:
- ❖ None significant
  - "in a bubble"

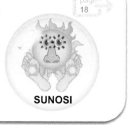

SUNOSI

Monoamine Oxidase Inhibitors (MAOIs)
"Chairman Mao"

❖ Antidepressants
❖ Parkinson's disease medications

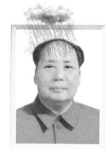

Monoamine Oxidase (MAO) is the enzyme that breaks down the **monoamine neurotransmitters**:

Serotonin (5-HT)　　　Norepinephrine (NE)　　　Dopamine (DA)

MAOI	Use	Year	Cost/mo	5-HT	NE	DA	MAO select-ivity *	Dietary tyramine risk	Wt gain	Sed-ation	Anti-cholin ergic	Rever-sible?
Tranylcypromine (PARNATE)	MDD	1961	$240	+++	+++	+++	A & B	++++	-	low	no	no
Isocarboxazid (MARPLAN)	MDD	1959	$780	+++	+++	+++	A & B	++++	-	low	no	no
Phenelzine (NARDIL)	MDD	1961	$43	+++	+++	+++	A & B	++++	++	low	no	no
Selegiline transdermal (EMSAM)	MDD	2006	$1650	++	++	+++	(A) & B	++	loss	low	no	no
Selegiline PO (ELDEPRYL)	Parkinson's	1989	$26	++	++	+++	B	+	loss	low	no	no
Rasagiline (AZILECT)	Parkinson's	2006	$270	++	++	+++	B	+	loss	low	no	no
Safinamide (XADAGO)	Parkinson's	2017	$780	+	+	+++	B	+/-	-	low	no	yes

MDD – Major Depressive Disorder; 5-HT – serotonergic; NE – noradrenergic; DA – dopaminergic

*Selectivity is dose dependent. Above recommended doses, selective MAO-B inhibitors can also inhibit MAO-A.

Monoamine Oxidase Inhibitors (MAOIs) are among the oldest antidepressants, available since 1959. The first MAOI (isocarboxazid) entered the market two years after the oldest TCA (imipramine, 1957). MAOIs are highly effective for treatment of depression, including cases resistant to modern antidepressants. MAOIs are particularly effective for "atypical depression", characterized by increased appetite, excessive sleep, fatigue, sensitivity to rejection, and moods that are highly reactive to circumstances.

"TIPS" – the MAOIs approved for depression:
► Tranylcypromine (PARNATE)
► Isocarboxazid (MARPLAN)
► Phenelzine (NARDIL)
► Selegiline transdermal (EMSAM)

The three oral MAOIs approved for treatment of depression in the U.S. are *irreversible* inhibitors of both MAO-A and MAO-B. Strict dietary restrictions are necessary to avoid the "cheese effect" of hypertensive crisis described in the isocarboxazid monograph, which is also applicable to phenelzine and tranylcypromine. Half-life for these MAOIs is irrelevant because inhibition of MAO is irreversible, with effect continuing for up to two weeks after the medication is discontinued.

In a simplified sense, MAO-A is more responsible for breaking down 5-HT and NE, while MAO-B is more specific for DA. For treatment of Parkinson's disease, MAO-B needs to be blocked. For treatment of depression, MAO-A needs to be blocked (to enhance 5-HT and NE), and blocking MAO-B may also be helpful (to enhance DA). In some countries, safer reversible inhibitors of monoamine oxidase A (RIMAs) are available for treatment of depression. Selective MAOIs available in the US block MAO-B for treatment of Parkinson's disease, and only one of these is reversible—safinamide (Xadago).

Due to risk of serotonin syndrome, all serotonergic medications are contraindicated with MAOIs. A washout period is necessary when switching to an MAOI, dependent on the half-life of the serotonergic agent (SSRI, SNRI, etc). As a rule of thumb, a drug clears the body after 5 half-lives. Wait at least 5 weeks after stopping fluoxetine (Prozac), which has a long half-life of 1 week. For the other SSRIs, wait two weeks after stopping the SSRI to start the MAOI.

A few antidepressants are safe to pair with MAOIs, including bupropion, trazodone, and those TCAs with minimal serotonergic activity such as nortriptyline, desipramine, maprotiline and trimipramine (Thomas and Shin, 2015)— "Non-Disparaged MOAI Tagalongs".

It is recommended that MAOIs be discontinued at least 10 days prior to elective surgery to avoid potentially fatal interactions with anesthetic agents.

Very serious dynamic interactions with serotonergic medications and tyramine-rich foods

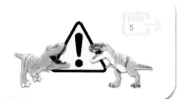

1959
$262–$286

Isocarboxazid (MARPLAN)
eye so kar BOX a zid / MAR plan
"Ice box Mars plan"

❖ Monoamine Oxidase Inhibitor
 – Irreversible MAOI
 – MAO-A & MAO-B
 – 5-HT > NE > DA

10
mg

FDA-approved for:
❖ Depression

> The following information applies to all of the non-selective MAO inhibitors used for treatment of depression —"TIP"
>
> ▶ **T**ranylcypromine (PARNATE)
> ▶ **I**socarboxazid (MARPLAN)
> ▶ **P**henelzine (NARDIL)

Patients taking MAOIs (with the exception of the low strength EMSAM patch) must <u>avoid tyramine-rich foods</u>. The list of forbidden foods is long. Failure to adhere to a low tyramine diet may lead to what was originally called the "cheese effect", a potentially fatal <u>hypertensive crisis</u>.

Tyramine = "Tire Rim"

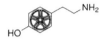

Tyramine is broken down by monoamine oxidase (MAO), which by definition MAOIs block. Without functioning MAO enzymes, tyramine accumulates and raises blood pressure.

The "tire rim" mnemonic can keep you from confusing tyramine with the amino acid tyrosine.

Note that if a patient is taking an oral MAOI for depression, phenelzine (Nardil) is the most likely prescription. Isocarboxazid (Marplan) scripts are exceedingly rare—it is <u>the least prescribed of all antidepressants</u>.

Dosing: Target dose is 20–60 mg/day divided BID–QID: Start 10 mg BID; May increase by 10 mg/day every 2–4 days; Max is 60 mg/day (20 mg TID or 30 mg BID); Taper gradually to stop.

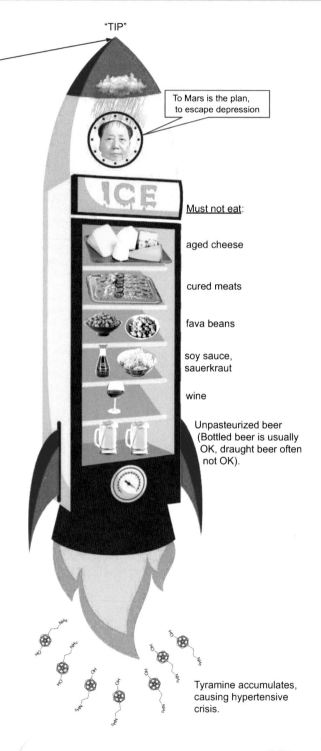

"TIP"

To Mars is the plan, to escape depression

ICE

<u>Must not eat</u>:

aged cheese

cured meats

fava beans

soy sauce, sauerkraut

wine

Unpasteurized beer (Bottled beer is usually OK, draught beer often not OK).

Tyramine accumulates, causing hypertensive crisis.

Dynamic interactions
❖ Serotonergic (strong) - contraindicated with other serotonergics
❖ Blocks tyramine breakdown (food interaction)
❖ Anticholinergic (mild)
❖ Hypertensive effects

Kinetic interactions
❖ None significant– "in a bubble"

MAOI

page 18

1961
$25–$86

Phenelzine (NARDIL)
FEN el zeen / NAR dil

"Gnarly Funnel"

- ❖ Monoamine Oxidase Inhibitor
  - – Irreversible MAOI
  - – MAO-A & MAO-B
  - – 5-HT > NE > DA

15 mg

FDA-approved for:
- ❖ Depression

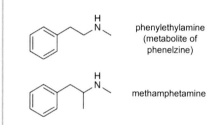

How could I be depressed while wearing this (g)narly phunnel?

Phenelzine is the least expensive ($43 monthly) and most commonly prescribed of the oral MAOIs for depression, although prescriptions for any MAOI are rare due to risk of serotonin syndrome and hypertensive crisis. Dietary tyramine must be restricted, as shown in the isocarboxazid (Marplan) monograph on the preceding page.

Phenelzine inhibits MAO-A and MAO-B almost equally, with slight preference for MAO-A. It is metabolized to phenylethylamine (PEA), which produces effects similar to a short acting amphetamine.

"Does this phunnel make me look phat?"– Unlike the other MAOIs, phenelzine may cause weight gain.

Risk of mortality in single-drug overdose with MAOIs is similar to that of tricyclics. Of 392 single-drug exposures to phenelzine reported to Poison Control, there were 2 deaths (Nelson & Spyker, 2017).

Dosing: Start 15 mg TID and rapidly increase to 30 mg TID (which is the maximum dose of 90 mg/day) then decrease slowly over several weeks to the lowest effective dose. Use lower dose with elderly patients. Taper slowly to stop.

phenylethylamine (metabolite of phenelzine)

methamphetamine

Dynamic interactions
- ❖ Serotonergic (strong) – contraindicated with other serotonergics
- ❖ Blocks tyramine breakdown (food interaction)
- ❖ Anticholinergic (mild)
- ❖ Hypertensive effects

MAOI

page 18

Kinetic interactions
- ❖ None significant
  - – "in a bubble"

1961
$187–$588

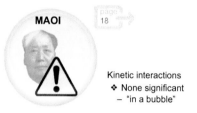

racemic mix

Tranylcypromine (PARNATE)
tran yl CY pro meen / PAR nate

"(Mao's) Trans prom Partner"

- ❖ Monoamine Oxidase Inhibitor
  - – Irreversible MAOI
  - – MAO-A & MAO-B
  - – DA & NE releaser
  - – 5-HT > NE > DA

10 mg

FDA-approved for:
- ❖ Depression

Tranylcypromine was released in 1961, the same year as phenelzine. Tranylcypromine has a short elimination half-life of 2.5 hours. The half-life is irrelevant, because inhibition of MAO is irreversible and the effect continues for up to 2 weeks after the medication is discontinued.

Dietary tyramine restriction is necessary to avoid hypertensive crisis, as depicted in the isocarboxazid (Marplan) monograph.

Risk of serious outcome from a single-drug overdose of tranylcypromine is about 40%, which is one of the highest morbidity rate among antidepressants. There was 1 death out of 330 single-drug overdoses (Nelson & Spyker, 2017).

Dosing: Start: 10 mg TID; After 2 weeks may increase by 10 mg/day q 1–3 weeks; Max is 60 mg/day (20 mg TID); Taper gradually to stop.

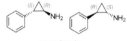

It don't matter that you're short.

Short half-life but this is irrelevant because inhibition of MAO is irreversible

Dynamic interactions
- ❖ Serotonergic (strong) – contraindicated with other serotonergics
- ❖ Blocks tyramine breakdown (food interaction)
- ❖ Anticholinergic (mild)
- ❖ Hypertensive effects

MAOI

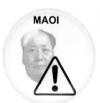

page 18

Kinetic interactions
- ❖ None significant
  - – "in a bubble"

Selegiline transdermal (EMSAM)

se LE ji leen / EM sam

"YosEmite Sam Seals gills"

❖ Monoamine Oxidase
Inhibitor
– MAO-B > MAO-A
– DA > NE > 5-HT

6
9
12
mg

FDA-approved for:

❖ Depression

Oral selegiline, at doses used for treatment of Parkinson's disease, is a selective inhibitor of MAO-B, which breaks down dopamine (DA). Oral selegiline at recommended doses does not inhibit MAO-A, making it ineffective for depression. It is necessary to block MAO-A to keep norepinephrine and serotonin from being broken down (oxidized).

The transdermal formulation of selegiline (EMSAM) allows the drug to achieve higher levels in the brain (where MAO-A breaks down serotonin) than in the gut (where MAO-A breaks down dietary tyramine).

Transdermal selegiline is the only MAOI available in the US for the treatment of depression that does not require dietary tyramine restriction at the clinically effective daily dose of 6 mg However, at higher doses, dietary restriction of tyramine is recommended.

Metabolism of selegiline produces a tiny amount of methamphetamine, which blocks dopamine reuptake and may contribute to the antidepressant benefit. The methamphetamine metabolite may produce a false positive on drug screens. Selegiline is not a controlled substance.

Selegiline is associated with a slight weight loss, which would be expected for something that is metabolized to methamphetamine.

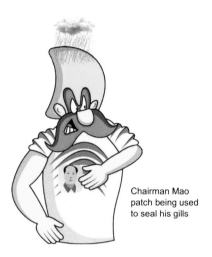

Chairman Mao patch being used to seal his gills

Dosing: Start with 6 mg patch QD; may increase strength by 3 mg QD in 2-week intervals; Max is 12 mg patch/24 hours. Dietary tyramine restriction is recommended above 6 mg. Taper to discontinue.

$41–
$150

Selegiline (ELDEPRYL)

se LE ji leen / ELD e pril

"Elderly Seal's gills"

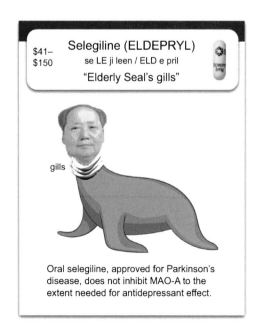

gills

Oral selegiline, approved for Parkinson's disease, does not inhibit MAO-A to the extent needed for antidepressant effect.

selegiline   methamphetamine

Dynamic interactions
❖ Serotonergic (strong) – contraindicated with other serotonergics
❖ Blocks tyramine breakdown (food interaction)
❖ Anticholinergic (mild)
❖ Hypertensive effects

Kinetic interactions
❖ 2B6 substrate

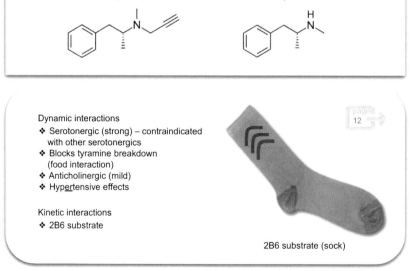

page 12

2B6 substrate (sock)

Cafer's Psychopharmacology | cafermed.com

Chapter 6 – Other Medications for Depression

2010
$172–$225 Deplin
$30–$45 MethylPro
$18–$25 other generics
$2–$12 folic acid

L-Methylfolate (DEPLIN)
meth il FO late / DEP lin
"Deep in My foliage"

❖ "Medical food" for depression
❖ Biologically active form of folate

7.5
15
mg

FDA-approved for:
❖ Augmentation of an antidepressant

Used off-label for:
❖ MTHFR deficiency

Folate (Vitamin B9), also known as folic acid, is necessary for synthesis of neurotransmitters including dopamine, norepinephrine, and serotonin. L-methylfolate is the active form of folate that crosses the blood-brain barrier with no need for enzymatic conversion.

About 1 in 3 individuals have difficulty converting folate to methylfolate due to a deficiency of the MTHFR enzyme (methylene tetrahydrofolate reductase). Among individuals with depression, about 60% have MTHFR mutations (Mischoulon et al, 2012). The 10% of individuals with 2 copies of the C677T MTHFR allele—"poor M*TH**F***Rs"—should be taking L-methylfolate.

Deplin is the brand of L-methylfolate marketed to physicians as a prescription-only "medical food" for depression. Other brands of L-methylfolate are now available without a prescription, though they are not FDA-regulated. There is no reason to believe Deplin is of higher quality than MethylPro, a reputable OTC version of L-methylfolate. Insurance rarely covers either brand, so the expense is borne out-of-pocket. Deplin costs 5x more than MethylPro and 50x more than generic folic acid.

L-methylfolate is intended to be an augmenting agent (add-on) to an antidepressant) in individuals who are not necessarily folate deficient. Refer to the "steps" advertisement below. As an augmenting agent, the number needed to treat with L-methylfolate was 6 (Papakostas et al, 2012).

Now that affordable brands are available, L-methylfolate is recommended over folic acid because it is more likely to be effective. There are no head-to-head trials of L-methylfolate vs folic acid, but results of L-methylfolate trials were more impressive.

Obese patients are more likely to respond to L-methylfolate, possibly because obesity causes inflammation, which impedes serotonin production (Shelton et al, 2015; *The Carlat Psychiatry Report*, Aug 2019). Generic folic acid may be adequate for non-obese individuals with normal MTHFR genes.

Supplementation of an antidepressant (fluoxetine specifically) with **generic folic acid** 0.5 mg/day demonstrated modest benefit at 10 weeks of treatment (Coppen & Bailey, 2000). The effect size was small, and some studies have not shown benefit from folate augmentation of antidepressants. Regardless, adding folate (vitamin B9) is a *benign* intervention—*folate is "Vitamin Be-nign"*.

Some studies combined folate (vitamin B9) with vitamins B6 and B12, Count by 3's—B6, B9, B12 = pyridoxine, folate, and cobalamin, respectively. Folic acid (B9) supplements can mask megaloblastic anemia that would otherwise lead to a diagnosis of vitamin B12 (cobalamin) deficiency. If untreated, B12 deficiency leads to peripheral neuropathy.

EnLyte is another prescription-only medical food containing 7 mg of L-methylfolate 7 mg and other "brain-ready, pre-metabolized coenzymes and cofactors". It costs about $170 monthly.

Folate is present in fresh green vegetables and other sources listed below. Garbanzo beans (chickpeas) contains an abundance of folate. Cooking reduces folate content by as much as 90%.

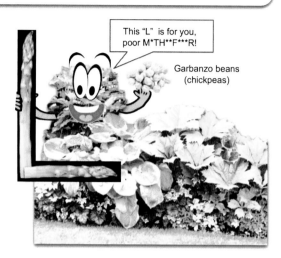

This "L" is for you, poor M*TH**F***R!

Garbanzo beans (chickpeas)

Now let's talk about actual folate deficiency. About 20% of depressed patients have low folate levels. Individuals with low folate do not respond as well to antidepressants. Patients with normal serum folic acid levels may still respond to treatment with folate because levels in the CNS may be low.

Folate deficiency leads to an elevation of homocysteine, a nonessential amino acid. Homocysteine is an NMDA receptor agonist and oxidant, i.e., something damaging to human cells An elevated homocysteine level is associated with cardiovascular disease.

No homo!

Folic acid deficiency during pregnancy leads to neural tube defects.

Dosing: For Deplin (expensive, prescription) or MethylPro (affordable, OTC) start 7.5 mg QD and increase to 15 mg, which is the target and maximum dose. MethylPro is available in 2.5, 5, 7.5, 10, 15 mg capsules. For generic folic acid (cheap) to augment an antidepressant you would give 0.5–5 mg QD. To treat folic acid deficiency, use 1 mg daily of generic folic acid plus a multivitamin. For a patient who responds to L-methylfolate for depression, consider changing to folic acid 3 mg (cheaper) at 6 months and see if recovery is maintained (Chris Aiken, MD, *The Carlat Psychiatry Report*, Aug 2019).

> **FOLINIC acid** is a similar supplement, which may be better (than L-methylfolate) for individuals who do not have MTHFR mutations. Folinic acid has advantages over the other forms of folate for those with folate receptor-alpha autoantibodies.

From a Deplin advertisement:

Deplin®
Partial Response
Antidepressant
Depression

Top sources of folate in food:
#1 Garbanzo beans (chickpeas)
#2 Liver
#3 Pinto beans
#4 Lentils
#5 Spinach
#6 Asparagus
#7 Avocado
#8 Beets
#9 Black eyed peas
#10 Broccoli

Dynamic interactions:
❖ None significant

Kinetic interactions:
❖ Valproic acid and other anticonvulsants can deplete folate levels. This is unlikely to be relevant for medication management involving Deplin.

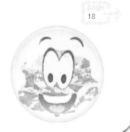

page 18

Ketamine (KETALAR)
KET a meen / KET a lar
"Cat (is) taller (than) Cat tamer"

❖ NMDA receptor antagonist
❖ Dissociative anaesthetic
❖ DEA Schedule III

FDA-approved for:
❖ General anesthesia

Used off-label for:
❖ Treatment-resistant depression
❖ Agitation in emergency department or ambulance
❖ Refractory chronic pain

Ketamine (Ketalar) is a dissociative anaesthetic that has shown rapid efficacy in relieving refractory depression following intravenous infusion. It is not FDA-approved for this indication but is increasingly utilized as an alternative to electroconvulsive therapy (ECT).

Ketamine's rapid antidepressant effect has been demonstrated by over 20 controlled trials. The effects of ketamine on depression are apparent as early as 40 minutes after infusion and are maintained for at least 2–3 days. Within two hours of ketamine treatment, patients are generally lucid and not sedated. By four hours, there appears to be continued improvement in positive thinking and hopefulness. By one week after a single infusion, depressive symptoms are likely to recur to some extent.

Side effects of ketamine include dissociation, visual hallucinations, sialorrhea (hypersalivation), nausea, vertigo, tachycardia, and elevated blood pressure. Serious risks include increased intracranial and intraocular pressure. Unlike other general anesthetics, ketamine does not suppress respiratory drive, which makes it great for anesthesia in third world countries. However, there is a possibility of laryngospasm [luh RING go spaz um], sudden involuntary contraction of vocal cords that can be fatal via suffocation. Catastrophic outcomes are rare when ketamine is used at subanesthetic antidepressant doses, but the patient needs to be monitored with emergency services available.

Ketamine has a black box warning of a 12% risk of emergence reactions (as in emerging from general anesthesia) varying in severity from pleasant dream-like states to hallucinations, or delirium. This may manifest as confusion, excitement, or irrational behavior. The duration of an emergence reaction is usually a few hours, with recurrences up to 24 hours post-op in some cases, but with no residual psychological effects.

The presumed antidepressant mechanism of ketamine is NMDA receptor antagonism, which reduces the activity of glutamate, the brain's most important excitatory neurotransmitter. The mechanism appears to somehow involve the endogenous opioid system (endorphins). Ketamine is not an opioid, but when naltrexone (opioid antagonist) was administered prior to a ketamine infusion, ketamine was ineffective for depression (Williams NR et al, 2018). Naltrexone does not block the dissociative effect of ketamine. Benzodiazepines and Z-drugs (zolpidem, etc) can attenuate the antidepressant effect of ketamine, so they should be washed out prior to treatment.

Originally synthesized from phencyclidine (PCP, "angel dust"), ketamine is a Schedule III controlled substance with potential for abuse and psychological dependence. Ketamine has a half-life of 10–15 minutes, which is shorter than other dissociatives such as PCP and dextromethorphan. The total dissociative experience should last no longer than 1–2 hours.

Recreational users of "special K" can snort, inject, or take it orally. The desired recreational effects include euphoria, derealization, visual hallucinations, and increasing awareness of sound and color. A bad experience from too much ketamine is referred to as falling into a "K-hole", where the user feels trapped in a frozen state, as if stuck in a hole peering out, detached from their physical presence. While stuck in a "K-hole", the user can, for instance, think about moving their arm and then see an arm moving in front of them, but the association between the thought and the movement does not register.

Risks with long-term maintenance treatment of depression with ketamine are unknown. Studies in mice suggest the potential for irreversible cognitive decline with chronic use (Ding et al, 2016).

Dosing: For treatment-resistant depression, the optimal ketamine protocol has not been clearly established. The most common frequency is twice weekly infusions for up to 4 weeks using a relatively low dose of 0.5 mg/kg administered over 40 minutes. Compare this to the anesthetic dose of 1–4.5 mg/kg—also the IV/IM dose used for agitation in the ambulance or emergency department.

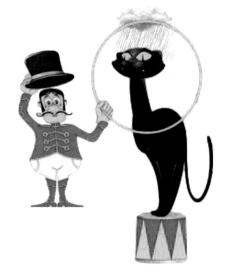

Ketamine is an alternative to:

▶ Electroconvulsive therapy (ECT)
▶ Transcranial magnetic stimulation (TMS)
▶ Deep brain stimulation (DBS)

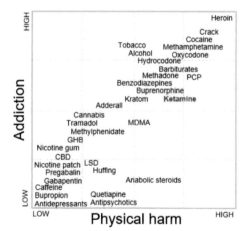

Physical harm is subjectively applied, as we are not comparing apples to apples. Since tobacco is responsible for 20% of deaths in the US, one could reasonably argue its relative harm is understated.

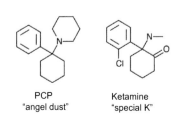

PCP
"angel dust"

Ketamine
"special K"

Dynamic interactions:
❖ Naltrexone can block the antidepressant effect of ketamine.
❖ Benzodiazepines and Z-drugs make ketamine less effective for depression.
❖ Hypertension
❖ Sedation

Kinetic interaction:

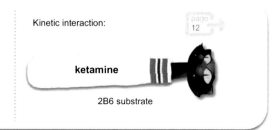

ketamine

2B6 substrate

Esketamine (SPRAVATO)
es KET a meen / sprah VAH toe
"Scat tamer – Spray gato"

❖ NMDA receptor antagonist
❖ Dissociative drug
❖ DEA Schedule III

56
84
mg

FDA-approved for:
❖ Treatment-resistant depression

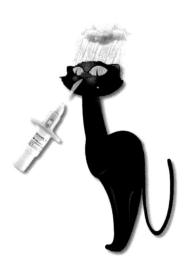

Ketamine (racemic)

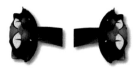

esketamine
(S) enantiomer

more of an
anaesthetic

arketamine
(R) enantiomer

more of a
hallucinogen

Esketamine nasal spray (Spravato) is the first novel antidepressant approved (2019) in over three decades. Esketamine is indicated for treatment-resistant depression (TRD) in conjunction with an oral antidepressant. It was developed for commercial purposes because the patent for ketamine was long expired.

As the name would suggest, esketamine is the S-enantiomer of ketamine, which has been increasingly used off-label for TRD. Like racemic ketamine, esketamine is a Schedule III controlled substance.

It is unknown whether the antidepressant action of the S-enantiomer is superior, inferior, or equal to racemic ketamine. The opposite enantiomer, R-ketamine (arketamine) is also under investigation. S-ketamine is more responsible for the anesthetic effect, while R-ketamine is more responsible for hallucinations because it is 3–4 times more potent at blocking NMDA receptors than R-ketamine. S-ketamine appears to be less effective than R-ketamine at reducing depressive symptoms (Stahl, 2015) but may be less likely to cause psychoactive side effects.

The induction phase for Spravato is twice weekly over 4 weeks, then weekly x 4, then every 1–2 weeks for maintenance treatment. It costs about $625 per dose.

Spravato is less convenient than would be expected for a nasal spray. It must be given in the presence of a health care provider and should never be dispensed to the patient for home use. The patient must be observed for 2 hours and cannot drive for the rest of the day. Due to the risk of vomiting, the patient must fast for 2 hours (no fluid for 30 minutes) prior to treatment.

Most of the therapeutic effect of esketamine is apparent by 24 hours after the first dose. Up to 75% of patients experience dissociation with Spravato. None of the clinical trials were controlled for the dramatic "high" esketamine produces. It was well-tolerated, with only 5% of subjects dropping out within one year due to side effects.

8 to 17% of patients have elevated blood pressure > 40 mmHg or diastolic BP elevation > 20 mmHg. 3% of patients will have systolic blood pressure elevation to about 180 mmHg . Blood pressure elevation peaks 40 minutes after administration and lasts about 4 hours. Due to this risk, esketamine is contraindicated with arteriovenous malformation or aneurysmal vascular disease (including aortic, intracranial, and peripheral arterial vessels). Stimulants such as Adderall or Ritalin could increase the risk of BP elevation.

With an 18% drug-placebo separation in relapse rates, esketamine's long-term benefits appear comparable to those seen with augmentation of an antidepressant with an atypical antipsychotic (Borges et al, 2014; The Carlat Psychiatry Report, Jun/Jul 2019). Long term use past one year has not been tested for the potential of cognitive impairment.

Esketamine prescribers must register through a Risk Evaluation and Mitigation Strategy (REMS) program, and the DEA will do an in-person inspection of the provider's office.

For cost savings, generic ketamine can be put into an atomizer for intranasal delivery as off-label option for 1% of the cost of esketamine.

The two available strengths of esketamine are 56 mg and 84 mg. The 56 mg dose is supplied in two 28 mg vials, and the 84 mg dose in three 28 mg vials. Each vial is delivered by 2 sprays, one in each nostril. Therefore 56 mg is delivered by 4 total sprays, and 84 mg by 6 total sprays. Wait 5 minutes between each 28 mg vial. Check BP before each dose and 40 minutes afterwards. Weigh risk/benefit if pre-treatment BP is > 140/90.

Dosing: The first dose should be 56 mg. Subsequent doses can be either 56 mg or 84 mg, depending on response and tolerability. Treatment is 2x/wk for first 4 weeks (8 treatments), then once weekly for the next 4 weeks (4 treatments), then every 1–2 weeks thereafter.

NMDA receptor

glutamate in
glutamate
binding site

binding site for:
❖ memantine
❖ amantadine
❖ ketamine
❖ PCP

glycine in
glycine
binding site

extracellular

intracellular

Ca²⁺ channel

NMDA receptors are involved in synaptic plasticity and memory. Lightly blocking the receptor is neuroprotective. However, if the receptor is blocked completely, neurons cannot function. The street drug PCP, aka "angel dust", strongly blocks NMDA receptors, causing psychosis. Ketamine is weaker than PCP, but strong enough to cause anaesthesia and dissociation. Memantine (Namenda) is an Alzheimer's medication that blocks the NMDA receptor just enough to improve memory.

Dynamic interactions:
❖ Naltrexone can block the antidepressant effect of ketamine.
❖ Benzodiazepines and Z-drugs make ketamine less effective.
❖ Hypertension
❖ Sedation

Kinetic interaction:

page 12

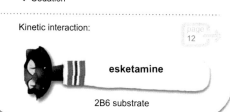

esketamine

2B6 substrate

Brexanolone (ZULRESSO)
brex AN oh lone / zul RESS o

"Zulu resigns (to) Brex (feed) alone"

Allopregnanolone

❖ Neurosteroid for
postpartum depression

FDA-approved for:
❖ Postpartum depression

In 2019, the first two novel antidepressants in over three decades were approved—esketamine (Spravato) and brexanolone (Zulresso). Brexanolone is the first medication FDA-approved for postpartum depression. Brexanolone is a synthetic version of allopregnanolone ("*all pregnant and alone*"), an endogenous neurosteroid made from progesterone that is increased during pregnancy.

It is theorized that withdrawal from allopregnanolone after childbirth can lead to postpartum depression and anxiety. Conventional antidepressants are known to raise levels of endogenous allopregnanolone.

Brexanolone acts at the GABA-A receptor complex, as do several classes of drugs that calm down the central nervous system, including benzodiazepines and barbiturates (see below). Unsurprisingly for something that works through the GABA-A receptor, brexanolone has anxiolytic, sedative, and anticonvulsant properties.

Brexanolone is insultingly expensive and must be given as an IV infusion over 60 hours! The cost of the drug is $34,000 not including the cost of hospitalization.

The advantage of brexanolone is speed of symptom improvement. Roughly 75% of patients reported at least a 50% reduction in depressive symptoms. Remission of depression may occur within a couple of days. 94% of patients who responded maintained their response at one month. Not bad!

It appears to be safe with breastfeeding—"*Brex (feed) alone*". The infant receives only 1–2% of maternal weight-adjusted dose. Excessive sedation is possible, so another adult should be present during treatment when mom has the baby. So you're technically not supposed to brexfeed *alone* on brexanolone.

Oral brexanolone is in development.

Allopregnanolone balance may play a role in other psychiatric disorders. Low levels are associated with depression and PTSD. High levels are also associated with depression, as well as anxiety and irritability (Bäckström et al, 2014).

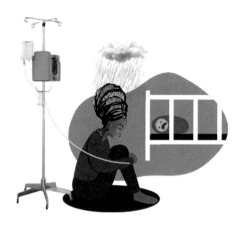

Dosing: Given intravenously over 60 hours; Start 30 mcg/kg/hr for 4 hours, then 60 mcg/kg/hr for 20 hours then 90 mcg/kg/hr for 28 hours, then 60 mcg/kg/hr for 4 hours, then 30 mcg/kg/hr for 4 hours = 60 hours total

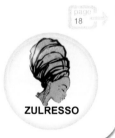

page 18 →

Dynamic interactions:
❖ Sedation / CNS depression

Kinetic interactions:
❖ No relevant kinetic interactions - "in a bubble"

ZULRESSO

GABA(A) receptor

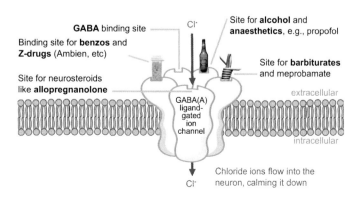

GABA binding site

Binding site for **benzos** and **Z-drugs** (Ambien, etc)

Site for neurosteroids like **allopregnanolone**

Cl⁻

Site for **alcohol** and **anaesthetics**, e.g., propofol

Site for **barbiturates** and meprobamate

extracellular

GABA(A) ligand-gated ion channel

intracellular

Chloride ions flow into the neuron, calming it down

Cl⁻

GABA receptor ligands

GABA(A) agonists
❖ Alcohol
❖ Ativan, alprazolam, etc (benzos)
❖ Amytal, etc (barbiturates)
❖ Ambien, etc (Z-drugs)
❖ Anesthetics
❖ Allopregnanolone (brexanolone)

GABA(A) antagonist
❖ Flumazenil (Romazicon) at the benzodiazepine site

GABA(B) agonists
❖ Baclofen (antispasmodic)
❖ GHB (Xyrem)

Note that gabapentin (Neurontin) and pregabalin (Lyrica) have chemical structures similar to GABA but they do **not** bind GABA receptors.

hypericin   hyperforin

St John's Wort (SJW)

Hypericum perforatum

St John's "wart"

SJW
$7–$35

❖ Herbal antidepressant

300
350
450
500
700
900
1000
mg

FDA-approved for:
❖ N/A

Effective for:
❖ Mild depression

Possibly effective for:
❖ Menopausal symptoms
❖ Social anxiety
❖ Somatoform disorders

St John's wort (SJW) is an OTC herbal antidepressant. SJW has demonstrated superiority to placebo for treatment of <u>mild depression</u>. It is considered ineffective for moderate to severe depression. Most psychiatrists do not recommend it, although psychiatrists are rarely consulted for mild depression.

The only advantage of SJW is obtainability without a doctor's order. The main drawback is potential for drug-drug <u>interactions</u>.

As with any herbal supplement, St John's wort contains many chemicals. It is not entirely clear which are responsible for the antidepressant effect, but <u>hypericin</u> (about 0.3% of the extract) is likely involved. The primary phytochemical constituent of St John's wort is hyperforin (about 3%). The composition of various chemicals may vary greatly between brands.

The likely mechanism of SJW is <u>serotonin reuptake inhibition</u>, like many prescription antidepressants. It also inhibits reuptake of norepinephrine and dopamine. It also has potent affinity for the adenosine, serotonin 5HT1, benzodiazepine and γ-aminobutyric acid (GABA) receptors. Plus, it may weakly inhibit monoamine oxidase. Lots of chemicals, lots of pharmacologic effects.

There is no FDA-approved indication for SJW. In 2000, the FDA issued a warning that SJW can <u>reduce the serum levels of many drugs</u> through in<u>D</u>uction of CYP450 enzymes.

Side effects of SJW are generally mild and may include insomnia, vivid dreams, irritability and GI discomfort. At high doses it may cause <u>phototoxic</u> skin reactions. It is not recommended to combine SJW with antidepressants due to risk of serotonin syndrome.

Hypericin is metabolized through the liver with half-life of about 25 hours.

St. John's wort is so named because it blooms near June 24th, the birthday of John the Baptist. "Wort" is an old English word for plant.

Dosing: 250 mg BID to 600 mg TID (Typically 300 mg TID). Products are generally standardized to contain 0.1–0.3% hypericin and/or 3–6% hyperforin

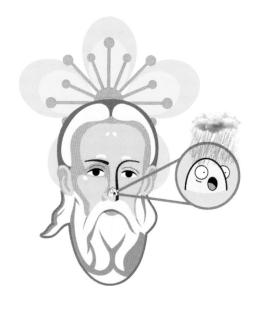

Hype<u>ric</u>in - *"Hyper rice"*

Hypericin may be the main chemical in St John's wort responsible for the antidepressant effect.

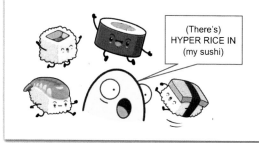

(There's) HYPER RICE IN (my sushi)

Dynamic interactions:
❖ Serotonergic
❖ Photosensitivity

Kinetic interactions:
❖ 1A2 inducer (major)
❖ 2C9 inducer (minor)
❖ 3A4 inducer (major)
❖ P-glycoprotein inducer (increased removal of P-gp substrates from the brain)

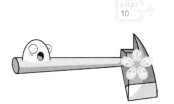

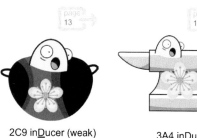

1A2 in<u>D</u>ucer

2C9 in<u>D</u>ucer (weak)

3A4 in<u>D</u>ucer

page 10

page 13

page 16

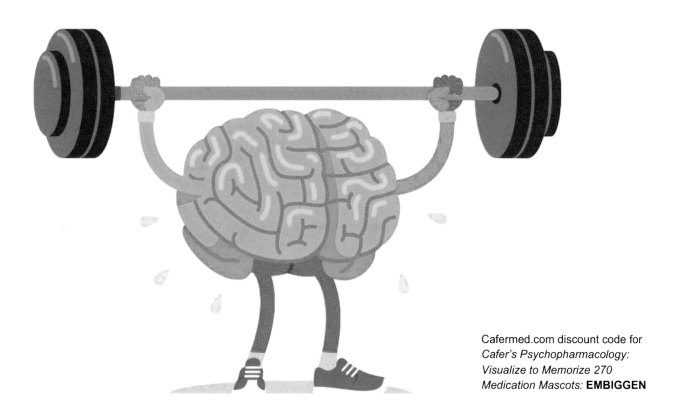

Cafermed.com discount code for
*Cafer's Psychopharmacology:
Visualize to Memorize 270
Medication Mascots:* **EMBIGGEN**

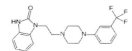

2015
$99–$427

Flibanserin (ADDYI)
fli BAN se rin / ADD ee

"Flibbin' Addicted (to love)"

❖ Norepinephrine-dopamine disinhibitor (NDDI)
❖ 5-HT$_{1A}$ agonist
❖ 5-HT$_{2A}$ antagonist

100 mg

FDA-approved for:

❖ Hypoactive Sexual Desire Disorder in premenopausal women

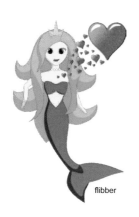

flibber

Flibanserin (Addyi), released in 2015, is FDA-approved for Hypoactive Sexual Desire Disorder in premenopausal women (it has not been tested in men or postmenopausal women). It was originally developed as an antidepressant.

Addyi has been colloquially referred to as the "female Viagra", but it has nothing in common with Viagra (sildenafil). Its mechanism involves dopamine, norepinephrine, and serotonin (5-HT).

	Viagra (sildenafil)	Addyi (flibanserin)
Mechanism	PDE inhibitor	5-HT$_{1A}$ agonist and 5-HT$_{2A}$ antagonist, which leads to increase of DA and NE activity
For use by	Men	Women
Purpose	Erection	Increased interest in sex
Response rate	80%	10% showed benefit over placebo
Effect size	Substantial improvement	Slight improvement
# scripts/year	> 2,000,000	About 5,000
Cost	$6 per tablet	$14 per tablet ($415/mo)
Instructions	PRN	Every day at HS
Contraindicated with	Nitroglycerine (hypotension)	Alcohol within 2 hours (hypotension); 3A4 inhibitors; Fluconazole (fluffer inHibitor of several relevant CYPs)
Other uses	Pulmonary arterial HTN	None

Physicians had to be certified to prescribe Addyi, but this restriction was lifted in 2019. Originally women taken Addyi were expected to abstain from alcohol because the combination can cause severe hypotension/syncope. In 2019 the contraindication with alcohol was softened. Addyi is contraindicated with liver impairment and with (strong to moderate) 3A4 inHibitors. These contraindications all relate to increased risk of hypotension/syncope and are all presented as black box warnings.

Women taking flibanserin reported an increase in "satisfying sexual events" from 2.8 to 4.5 events per month. Women taking placebo improved from 2.7 to 3.7 events per month.

Flibanserin has turned out to be a flop of a medication, with only about 5,000 annual prescriptions. Its lack of popularity is unsurprising given its disappointing efficacy, costs, and (previously) mandated alcohol abstinence pledge. In 2019 the label warning for alcohol use was softened to state "women should discontinue drinking alcohol at least two hours before taking Addyi at bedtime or skip the Addyi dose that evening. Women should not consume alcohol at least until the morning after taking Addyi at bedtime".

For context, blocking 5-HT$_{2A}$ is the opposite of what hallucinogens do. LSD is a 5-HT$_{2A}$ agonist. Second generation antipsychotics also block 5-HT$_{2A}$—*2A for 2nd gen Antipsychotic*.

Dosing: The starting and maintenance dose is 100 mg QD HS.

> **Flibanserin does not appear to contribute to serotonin syndrome.**

Comparison with other medications that can improve sexual functioning via serotonin receptors:

	Indication	5-HT$_{1A}$	5-HT$_{2A}$
Flibanserin (ADDYI)	Hypoactive sexual desire disorder	Agonist	(Antagonist)
Trazodone (DESYREL)	Depression (off-label for insomnia)	(Agonist)	Antagonist
Nefazodone (SERZONE)	Depression	(Agonist)	Antagonist
Buspirone (BUSPAR)	Anxiety	Partial agonist	-
Pimavanserin (NUPLAZID)	Hallucinations and delusions associated with Parkinson's	-	Inverse agonist

Dynamic interactions:
❖ Sedation/CNS depression
❖ Hypotensive
 - contraindicated with alcohol

Kinetic interactions:
❖ 3A4 substrate
 - contraindicated with moderate to strong 3A4 inHibitors, which may increase flibanserin levels, leading to hypotension.
❖ 2C9 substrate
❖ 2C19 substrate
❖ Contraindicated with fluconazole (Diflucan) which is a "fluffer" inHibitor of the 3 CYPs that metabolize flibanserin, causing 7-fold increase in flibanserin levels, leading to hypotension

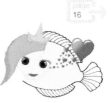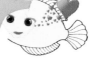

3A4 substrate

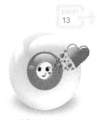

2C9 substrate

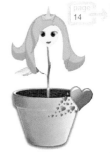

2C19 substrate

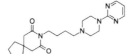

| #90
1986
$7–$62 | | Buspirone (BUSPAR)
BU spi rone / BU spar
"Bus spear" | ❖ Anxiolytic
❖ 5-HT$_{1A}$ serotonin receptor
   partial agonist
❖ Non-addictive | 5 mg
7.5
10
15
30 |

FDA-approved for:

❖ Anxiety

Used off-label for:

❖ Augmentation of SSRI for depression
❖ Antidepressant-associated sexual dysfunction
❖ SSRI-induced bruxism (tooth grinding)
❖ Movement disorders (high dose)
   - Tardive dyskinesia
   - Chorea
   - Levodopa induced dyskinesias
❖ Hostility in patients with cardiac impairment

Some of the generic multi-scored tablets look like yellow school buses. However, most generics buspirone tabs are white, and "school bus" is slang for a multi-scored yellow 2 mg alprazolam (Xanax) tablet.

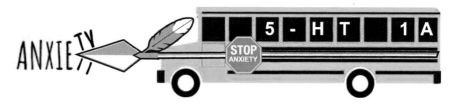

Buspirone (BuSpar) is a serotonin 5-HT$_{1A}$ receptor partial agonist (SRA) FDA-approved for generalized anxiety disorder (GAD). It is unrelated to other anxiolytics. Buspirone is non-addictive and generally non-sedating. Unlike other medications in this chapter, buspirone works in a slow and steady fashion, like an antidepressant. Contrast this with benzodiazepines, which work immediately but are addictive. Unlike benzodiazepines, buspirone is generally not useful as a PRN anxiolytic because optimum efficacy usually requires 2 to 4 weeks of regular administration. Some patients regard buspirone as an effective PRN, likely due to placebo effect.

"Buspar is benign." Buspirone is one of the safest psychotropic medications, with no need for laboratory monitoring. There are no absolute contraindications (other than allergy to buspirone). No deaths have been reported with single-drug overdose. It is generally well tolerated, but potential side effects include nausea, headache and jitters. It does not cause weight gain. Withdrawal is not an issue if buspirone is stopped without tapering.

"Buspirone doesn't have to be used alone!" (Madalyn Hoke, PA-S). Buspirone can be combined with practically any other psychotropic medication, with a couple of exceptions.

Buspirone is avoided with MAOIs, although there is evidence that buspirone does not cause serotonin syndrome (The scoop on serotonin syndrome; Foong et al; Canadian Pharmacists Journal, 2018)

> **Buspirone does not appear to cause serotonin syndrome.**

It is redundant to combine buspirone with vilazodone (Viibryd) because vilazodone has intrinsic 5-HT$_{1A}$ receptor partial agonist activity. Pharmacologically, *"Viibryd is like a hybrid"* of an SSRI and buspirone (page 57).

Buspirone is commonly prescribed along with an antidepressant, although caution is advised due to a small possibility of serotonin syndrome. An SSRI plus buspirone is good for anxiety, but there is better evidence for other augmenting agents for treatment-resistant depression (TRD). More effective adjuncts for

TRD include lithium, aripiprazole (Abilify), quetiapine (Seroquel), risperidone (Risperdal), and liothyronine (Cytomel—T3 thyroid hormone). However, buspirone is safer and better tolerated than these more proven adjuncts.

Unlike most serotonergics, buspirone may enhance sexual functioning. Buspirone shares some properties with flibanserin (Addyi), a 5-HT$_{1A}$ receptor agonist approved for hypoactive sexual desire disorder (page 73).

Buspirone can serve as an antidote for SSRI-induced bruxism (tooth grinding). Buspirone is used off-label at high dose for treatment of movement disorders including chorea, tardive dyskinesia and levodopa induced dyskinesias. It may improve cognitive functioning in schizophrenia and Alzheimer's disease. When used for anxiety with alcohol use disorder, it decreases drinking days (Kranzler et al, 1994).

"This school bus ain't for kids"—Although there are no safety issues, buspirone does not appear to be effective for treatment of GAD in individuals under age 18.

Buspirone has a short half-life of 2–3 hours, so it requires BID or TID dosing (usually TID). Although inconvenient, some patients prefer multiple daily dosing for better perceived control of symptoms. However, it is not expected to be immediately effective. Benefit is achieved gradually over 2–4 weeks, but placebo effect can be a powerful thing.

Dosing: Buspirone is typically started 7.5–10 mg BID or TID and titrated quickly to a target dose of 15 mg TID or 20 mg BID, with FDA maximum dose of 60 mg/day. Starting at 15 mg BID is ok. It is recommended to take buspirone consistently with food or consistently without food, because it is better absorbed when taken with meals. For off-label treatment of movement disorders, it may be necessary to titrate buspirone as high as 180 mg/day. A higher dose of buspirone will be needed if it is combined with a strong 3A4 inDucer such as carbamazepine (Tegretol). Unless the dose is very high, buspirone may be discontinued without tapering.

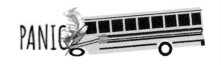

BuSpar was found to be ineffective for panic disorder.

Comparison with other medications that can improve sexual functioning via serotonin receptors:

Serotonergic medication	Indication	5-HT$_{1A}$	5-HT$_{2A}$
Flibanserin (ADDYI)	Hypoactive sexual desire	Agonist	(Antagonist)
Trazodone (DESYREL)	Depression/insomnia	(Agonist)	Antagonist
Nefazodone (SERZONE)	Depression	(Agonist)	Antagonist
Buspirone (BUSPAR)	Anxiety	Partial agonist	-
Pimavanserin (NUPLAZID)	Hallucinations and delusions associated with Parkinson's disease	-	Inverse agonist

Dynamic interactions:
❖ Serotonergic
❖ Sedative (weak)

Kinetic interactions:
❖ 3A4 substrate

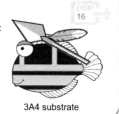

3A4 substrate

Meperidine (DEMEROL)

me PER i deen / DEM er ol

"Meeper Demoralized"

1942
$17 - $41

❖ Opioid
❖ Serotonergic
❖ Schedule II

50
100
mg

FDA-approved for:

❖ Moderate-to-severe pain

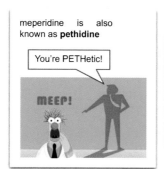

You are toxic and sedating. You should not be used at all.

Meperidine can certainly contribute to serotonin syndrome.

Meperidine (Demerol), also called pethidine, was the first synthetic opioid. Since it is synthetic, you would not refer to it as an opiate. Eduardo Fraifeld, MD opined that Demerol is "toxic and sedating" and "should not be used at all". Withdrawal symptoms are worse than with morphine. Meperidine should not be used for chronic pain. Its use for acute pain should be reserved for those allergic to first-line opioids. Oral administration is not advised due to extremely poor bioavailability. The usual route of administration is intramuscular (IM). It is not available for intravenous (IV) administration. Duration of action is very short, about 3 hours.

Meperidine is distinguished from other opioids by its serotonergic properties, caused by 5-HT reuptake inhibition. Meperidine was involved in a high-profile death from serotonin syndrome in 1984, which killed an 18-year-old college student named Libby Zion. The reaction occurred when meperidine was added to the MAOI phenelzine (Nardil).

Opioids, meperidine excluded, are potent pupillary constrictors. Due to meperidine's serotonergic and anticholinergic effects, it can cause dilation of pupils in some individuals. Withdrawal from meperidine manifests with dilated pupils like the other opioids. It is more likely than other opioids to cause seizures with overdose.

Although primarily a mu opioid receptor agonist, meperidine has more affinity for the kappa receptor than morphine, making meperidine more likely to cause dysphoria, hallucinations, and dissociation.

The metabolite of meperidine (normeperidine) is neurotoxic and may accumulate in cases of renal or hepatic impairment.

---

meperidine is also known as **pethidine**

You're PETHetic!

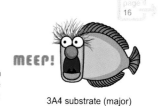

Dynamic interactions:

❖ Opioid agonist
  - Constipation
  - Sedation / CNS depression
  - Respiratory depression
  - Hypotension
❖ Lowers seizure threshold
❖ Prolongs QT interval
❖ Serotonergic (moderate)
❖ Anticholinergic
❖ Neurotoxicity

Kinetic interactions:

❖ Delayed gastric emptying
❖ 3A4 substrate
❖ Black box warning: concomitant use with 3A4 inhibitors or discontinuation of 3A4 inducers may cause fatal fentanyl concentration

3A4 substrate (major)

page 16

Causes of mydriasis and miosis

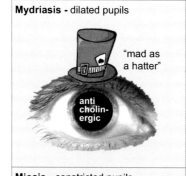

Mydriasis - dilated pupils

"mad as a hatter"

anti cholin- ergic

Sympathetic (fight or flight)	❖ Anticholinergics – atropine eye drops are highly anticholinergic and given for the purpose of dilating pupils for ophthalmologic exam	
With anticholinergic toxicity, also expect to see facial flushing.	❖ Antidepressants	
Mydriasis - "Oh *my*... what big eyes you have"	❖ Serotonin syndrome	
	❖ Stimulants	
Pronounced [mi DRAHY *uh* sis] or [mahy DRAHY *uh* sis]	❖ LSD, PCP, Hallucinogens	
	❖ Opioid withdrawal	
	❖ Meperidine (Demerol) - an opioid with anticholinergic and serotonergic properties	

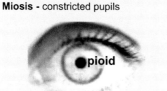

Miosis - constricted pupils

opioid

Parasympathetic (rest and digest)
Miosis - "*mini*-pupils"

❖ Opioids (other than meperidine) are the most potent pupillary constrictors
❖ Antipsychotics
❖ Trazodone (Desyrel) and mirtazapine (Remeron) – antidepressants with sedative properties
❖ Cholinergics, e.g., donepezil (Aricept)

Methadone (DOLOPHINE)

METH a dohn / DOLE o fene

"Dolphin's Method (to be) done" (using heroin)

1947
$12 - $41

❖ Long-acting opioid
❖ Schedule II

10 mg / ml

5
10
40 mg

FDA-approved for:

❖ Opioid dependence
❖ Chronic pain

Methadone (Dolophine), commonly used as maintenance treatment for heroin addiction, is a synthetic opioid with an exceptionally long half-life of 24 to 55 hours. Like other opioids, methadone is a Schedule II controlled substance. It has a 60 – 90% success rate for treating opioid use disorder (OUD), substantially more effective than abstinence-based treatment. This approach to addiction is considered "harm reduction" – the patient remains addicted to an opioid but avoids the social, health (overdose, dirty needles) and legal morbidity of using heroin. For short-acting opioids (heroin, morphine, oxycodone, etc) withdrawal symptoms may start within 6 – 8 hours from the last dose. The advantage of methadone is that withdrawal does not start until 24 hours.

Side effects are those typical of opioids. However, thanks to methadone's long half-life, tolerance to side effects develops quickly. So, with methadone there will be less persisting constipation, dizziness, sedation, nausea, and miosis compared other opioids Since methadone accumulates, the dose may need to be reduced after about 5 days to avoid toxicity.

The main risk of methadone is death by overdose due to respiratory depression. Methadone prolongs QT interval and increases risk for torsades de pointes at high dose.

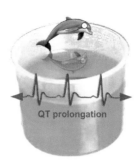

QT prolongation

Methadone, when used for opioid addiction (21-day detox or long-term maintenance) must only be dispensed by certified opioid treatment programs, under strict regulation. Originally, clinics had to dispense methadone in liquid form.

Methadone has weak serotonergic properties, making it a possible (but unlikely) contributor to serotonin syndrome when combined with antidepressants.

Methadone can contribute to serotonin syndrome.

Dynamic interactions:

❖ Opioid agonist
- Constipation
- Sedation / CNS depression
- Respiratory depression
- Hypotension
❖ Lowers seizure threshold
❖ Prolongs QT interval (moderate)
❖ Serotonergic (weak)

Kinetic interactions:

❖ Delays gastric emptying
❖ 2B6 substrate (major)
❖ 2C19 substrate
❖ 3A4 substrate
Black Box Warning: concomitant use with inhibitors of 3A4, 2B6, 2C19, 2C9, or 2D6 or discontinuation of concomitant inducers of these enzymes may cause potentially fatal respiratory depression.

3% of the population are 2B6 ultrarapid metabolizers (UMs). Methadone will be poorly effective for these individuals, and methadone may even be negative on standard drug screens.

page 12
page 14
page 16

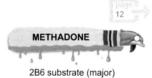

METHADONE

2B6 substrate (major)

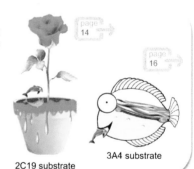

2C19 substrate

3A4 substrate

Fentanyl (DURAGESIC)

FEN ta nil / dur a GEES ik

"Fountain eel's Durable analgesic"

1984
$41 - $151

❖ Potent opioid
❖ Schedule II

FDA-approved for:

❖ Severe chronic pain

Fentanyl is a very high-potency opioid, dosed by mcg rather than mg. It is 100 times stronger than morphine. Recreational drugs (heroin, cocaine, etc.) may be laced with illegally-made fentanyl from China. Fentanyl is the most common cause of opioid overdose fatality. Fentanyl transdermal (Duragesic) is for opioid-tolerant patients only.

Fentanyl is weakly serotonergic. There are case studies of it causing serotonin syndrome when combined with an antidepressant.

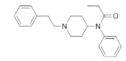

Opioids constrict pupils

Used patches are to be flushed down the toilet

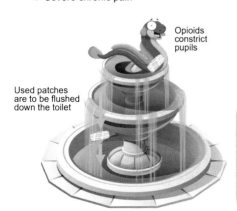

Dynamic interactions:

❖ Opioid agonist
- Constipation
- Sedation / CNS depression
- Respiratory depression
- Hypotension
❖ Lowers seizure threshold
❖ Serotonergic (weak)

Kinetic interactions:

❖ Delayed gastric emptying
❖ 3A4 substrate
❖ Black box warning: concomitant use with 3A4 inhibitors or discontinuation of 3A4 inducers may cause fatal fentanyl concentration

page 16

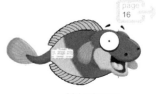

3A4 substrate

50 mg

Tramadol (ULTRAM)
TRAM a dol / UL tram
"Ultra ram Trauma doll"

#39
1995
IR: $7 - $41
ER: $32 - $123

Racemic mix

Pain medication
❖ Weak opioid
❖ SNRI
❖ DEA Schedule IV

FDA-approved for:
❖ Acute pain (mod to severe)
❖ Chronic pain (mod to severe) – ER formulation

Used off-label for:
❖ Fibromyalgia
❖ Premature ejaculation

Tramadol is a <u>partial (weak) agonist at the μ (mu) opioid receptor</u> with onset of pain relief in about 1 hour, with duration of about 6 hours. Tramadol is also a serotonin–norepinephrine reuptake inhibitor (SNRI) like venlafaxine (Effexor) and duloxetine (Cymbalta). Tramadol is not considered an antidepressant but may have some antidepressant and anxiolytic properties. Tramadol is not typically prescribed by psychiatrists. Tramadol can contribute to <u>serotonin syndrome if combined</u> with serotonergic antidepressants.

Tramadol was released in the US in 1995 and became a <u>Schedule IV</u> controlled substance in 2015 due to potential for abuse as an opioid. Compared to other opioids, respiratory depression and constipation are less of a problem with tramadol. With overdose, tramadol is more likely (than traditional opioids) to cause seizures than traditional opioids.

Side effects are similar to other opioids. In order of frequency, adverse effects occurring within 90 days included constipation (46%), nausea (40%), dizziness (33%), headache (32%), somnolence (25%), vomiting (17%), pruritus (11%) and psychiatric effects (14%). Tramadol has 8 black box warnings, comparable to other opioid medications.

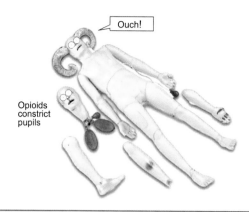
Ouch!

Opioids constrict pupils

Tramadol can contribute to serotonin syndrome.

Tramadol is available in a fixed dose combination with <u>ace</u>taminophen (Tylenol) called Ultra<u>cet</u>.

Dosing: The standard dose is 50 - 100 mg q4-6 hr PRN; Although it tends to be started at 50 mg, the label recommends to go slower "unless immediate onset is required" by starting 25 q AM; May increase by 25 mg/day in 3-day intervals to 25 mg q 6 hr PRN, then may increase by 50 mg in 3-day intervals to 50 mg q 6 hr PRN; <u>Maximum is 400 mg /day</u> (300 mg/day for > 75 years); use lowest effective dose and shortest effective treatment duration; To stop (if prolonged use), <u>taper slowly</u>, by no more than 10-25% in 2-4 week intervals.

Dynamic interactions:
❖ Opioid agonist
  - Constipation
  - Sedation / CNS depression
  - Respiratory depression
  - Hyp<u>o</u>tension
❖ Lowers seizure threshold
❖ QT prolongation
❖ Serotonergic

Kinetic interactions:
❖ Delays gastric emptying
❖ 3A4 substrate
❖ Tramadol is transformed by 2D6 to an active metabolite (desmethyltramadol) which is responsible for most of the opioid effect.
❖ Tramadol may be less effective for individuals with 2D6 poor metabolizer (PM) genotype (10% of population) or for individuals taking 2D6 inHibitors such as fluoxetine, paroxetine or bupropion.
❖ Black box warning: Respiratory depression and death have occurred in children with 2D6 ultra-rapid metabolizer (UM) genotype (5% of population).
❖ Black box warning: "Concomitant use or discontinuation of concomitant 3A4 inDucers, 3A4 inHibitors, or 2D6 inHibitors are complex; Such interactions require careful consideration of the effects on tramadol and its active metabolite".

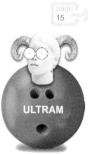

ULTRAM

2D6 prodrug

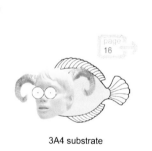
3A4 substrate

page 15
page 16

Tapentadol (NUCYNTA)
ta PENT a dol / Nu SEN ta
"Tap into doll's New scent"

Tapentadol does <u>not</u> appear to contribute to serotonin syndrome.

"The 'Nu' Tramadol" - tapentadol (Nucynta) was approved in 2009 for acute pain (moderate to severe) such as post-surgical pain. Tapentadol works as a mu opioid agonist and norepinephrine reuptake inhibitor (NRI). Tapentadol <u>does not significantly inhibit serotonin reuptake</u> like Tramadol does.

Tapentadol is a Schedule II controlled substance like traditional opioids such as morphine, oxycodone, hydrocodone, etc. Its actual opioid strength is weaker than oxycodone, and about equal to hydrocodone. Its (total) analgesic efficacy is about equivalent to oxycodone, with fewer gastrointestinal side effects. Nausea occurred about 50% of the time with tapentadol, compared to 70% with oxycodone.

The <u>label warns</u> not to combine tapentadol with serotonergic antidepressants, <u>but</u> in clinical trials patients took it concurrently with SSRIs without adverse effects.

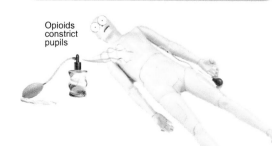
Opioids constrict pupils

Triptans for acute migraine headaches

Triptans are a family of tryptamine-based drugs used as abortive medication for migraines and cluster headaches. Triptans should be administered as quickly as possible upon headache onset. Early treatment decreases the likelihood of recurrence within 24 hours. The subcutaneous route is more effective but brings more side effects. Weakness or somnolence following triptan therapy may be part of the migraine attack, unmasked by the successful treatment of pain.

Longer-acting triptans such as naratriptan (Amerge) and frovatriptan (Frova) have a slower onset of action and lower initial response rate than other triptans, but they are better tolerated.

Triptans constrict blood vessels. They carry a small risk of heart attack, stroke, or seizure. All triptans are contraindicated with coronary artery disease, peripheral vascular disease, uncontrolled hypertension, history of stroke, or Wolff-Parkinson-White syndrome (extra electrical pathway in the heart with tachycardic episodes).

> **Triptans do not appear to cause serotonin syndrome.**

About 25% of triptan users are also prescribed an SSRI or SNRI. In 2006 the FDA issued a warning that triptans could contribute to serotonin syndrome when combined with SSRIs or SNRIs. The warning did not change prescribing practices, and the risk appears miniscule to nonexistent. Orlova et al (2018) estimated the risk at about one case of serotonin syndrome per 10,000 person-years of exposure to a triptan plus an SSRI/SNRI.

Serotonin syndrome is hypothesized to involve 5-HT_{1A} and 5-HT_{2A} receptors, while triptans are agonists at 5-HT_{1B} and 5-HT_{1D} receptors.

| #115
1992
$6–$112 | 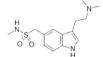 | **Sumatriptan (IMITREX)**
SOO ma TRIP tan / EM i trex
"Sumo tripped (in my tracks)" | ❖ Triptan for acute migraine
❖ 5-HT_{1B} receptor agonist
❖ 5-HT_{1D} receptor agonist | | 25
50
<u>100</u>
mg |

FDA-approved for:
- ❖ Migraine headache (acute)
- ❖ Cluster headache (acute)
  - subcutaneous route

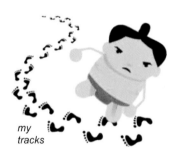

my tracks

Sumatriptan (Imitrex) is a triptan available via several methods of delivery. Subcutaneous administration is the most effective but brings more side effects than the PO route. Onset of migraine relief is within 30–60 minutes with oral formulation, 10 minutes with subcutaneous, and 10–15 minutes with nasal powder.

Elimination half-life of sumatriptan is about 2 hours. Side effects may include paresthesia, chest tightness, warm/cold sensation, vertigo, and fatigue. TREXIMET is a fixed-dose oral combination of sumatriptan with the NSAID naproxen.

Dosing: Oral sumatriptan is dosed 50–100 mg, may be repeated after 2 hours of PO or after 1 hour of SC dose. PO maximum of 200 mg/day. Subcutaneous dosing is 1–6 mg SC x 1, may repeat after 1 hour for max of 12 mg/day. With mild to moderate hepatic impairment, the PO max is 50 mg/dose. With severe hepatic impairment both PO and SC sumatriptan is contraindicated.

Dynamic interactions:
- ❖ Serotonergic, but highly unlikely to contribute to serotonin syndrome
- ❖ Hypertensive effects

Kinetic interactions:
- ❖ None significant

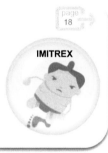

| #232
1998
$15–$186 | | **Rizatriptan (MAXALT)**
RYE za TRIP tan / MAX alt
"RZA tripped (on) Max altitude" | ❖ Triptan for acute migraine
❖ 5-HT_{1B} receptor agonist
❖ 5-HT_{1D} receptor agonist | | 5
<u>10</u>
mg |

FDA-approved for:
- ❖ Migraine headache (acute)

Unlike sumatriptan, rizatriptan (Maxalt) is not approved for cluster headaches and is not available by subcutaneous route.

Rizatriptan is metabolized by monoamine oxidase-A, which is inhibited by propranolol. Concomitant use with propranolol increases blood levels of rizatriptan by 70%.

No dosage adjustment is needed with hepatic impairment, which is an advantage of rizatriptan over sumatriptan.

Dosing: 5 or 10 mg PO, may be repeated in 2 hours.

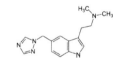

RZA of the Wu-Tang Clan, pronounced "rizza", while the medication is spelled "Riza" and pronounced [RYE-za]

Dynamic interactions:
- ❖ Serotonergic, but highly unlikely to contribute to serotonin syndrome
- ❖ Hypertensive effects

Kinetic interactions:
- ❖ Minimal, but propranolol increases plasma concentrations of rizatriptan by 70% by inhibiting monoamine oxidase-A

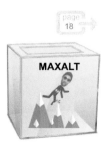

Centrally acting spasmolytics – "muscle relaxers"

Central muscle relaxants relieve muscle spasms through action in the central nervous system (CNS)—in the brainstem and spinal cord. They have no direct action on the contractile mechanism of muscles or the neuromuscular end plate.

Non-addictive spasmolytics

These centrally acting muscle relaxants are not controlled substances.

Muscle relaxant	cost/mo	Class	Details
Cyclobenzaprine (FLEXERIL)	$14	Tricyclic	#1 prescribed muscle relaxant. Structure is very similar to the TCA amitriptyline (Elavil). Cyclobenzaprine is a 5-HT$_2$ antagonist that works in the brainstem to reduce muscle tone by decreasing the activity of descending <u>serotonergic</u> neurons. Amitriptyline also does this.
Baclofen (LIORESAL)	$13	GABA(B) agonist	Baclofen is a derivative of the neurotransmitter GABA and works as a GABA(B) receptor agonist.
Methocarbamol (ROBAXIN)	$18	Carbamate	Methocarbamol lacks the abuse potential of the Schedule IV carbamate carisoprodol (Soma). It is also much safer.
Tizanidine (ZANAFLEX)	$17	Central alpha agonist	Same mechanism as clonidine (Catapres) and guanfacine (Tenex) with less antihypertensive effect.
Metaxalone (SKELAXIN)	$45	Oxazolidinone	Can contribute to <u>serotonin syndrome</u>; Most oxazolidinones are antibiotics, e.g., linezolid, which can also cause serotonin syndrome.
Orphenadrine (NORFLEX)	$42	Antihistamine/ anticholinergic	Structure very similar to diphenhydramine (Benadryl). Muscarinic antagonist and NMDA antagonist. Rarely prescribed.

Schedule IV spasmolytics

These centrally acting muscle relaxants are DEA Schedule IV controlled substances with potential for abuse and addiction.

Muscle relaxant	cost/mo	Class	Details
Meprobamate (MILTOWN)	$110	Carbamate	Was the most-prescribed anxiolytic in the pre-benzodiazepine era
Carisoprodol (SOMA)	$12	Carbamate	The prodrug of meprobamate (Miltown). Soma is the #3 most prescribed muscle relaxant (behind Flexeril and Robaxin), despite being addictive and dangerous.
Diazepam (VALIUM)	$9	Benzodiazepine	FDA-approved for anxiety, seizures, and muscle spasms.

1962
$40–$144

Metaxalone (SKELAXIN)
me TAX a lone / ska LAX in

"**Skel**etor Re**laxin**' (with a) **Meat ax, alone**"

❖ Antispasmodic
❖ CNS depressant
❖ Serotonergic

400
<u>800</u>
mg

FDA-approved for:
❖ Acute musculoskeletal pain

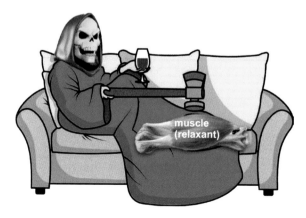

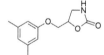

Our spooky mascots are generally reserved for antipsychotics, with Skelaxin as an exception.

> **Metaxalone <u>can</u> contribute to serotonin syndrome.**

The spasmolytic mechanism of metaxalone (Skelaxin) is unknown, other than being a general CNS depressant. It may be weak monoamine oxidase inhibitor (MAOI). If taken in large doses metaxalone may be sufficiently potent to cause <u>serotonin syndrome</u>.

Metaxalone is not commonly prescribed.

Dosing: For acute musculoskeletal pain, give 800 mg TID–QID on an empty stomach.

Dynamic interactions:

❖ Sedation/CNS depression
❖ Serotonergic (weak)

Kinetic interactions:

❖ Metabolized by seven different P450 enzymes (multi-CYP); Kinetic interactions occur but are unlikely to be clinically significant with so many Metabolic pathways—"in a box".

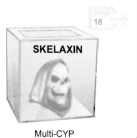

SKELAXIN

Multi-CYP

#46
1977
$2–$24

Cyclobenzaprine (FLEXERIL)
cy kloe BEN za preen / FLEX er il

"(tri) Cycle bends, Flexes 'n' rolls"

❖ Antispasmodic
❖ Tricyclic structure
❖ 5-HT$_2$ antagonist
❖ Non-controlled

5
7.5
<u>10</u>
mg

FDA-approved for:
❖ Muscle spasms

Used off-label for:
❖ Fibromyalgia
❖ Insomnia

Released in 1977, cyclobenzaprine (Flexeril) remains the #1 most prescribed muscle relaxant. It is <u>not a controlled substance</u>. Half-life is 18 hours, and it is generally dosed TID. Flexeril is modestly effective for acute lower back pain with muscle spasm, although <u>efficacy begins to decrease after about 4 days</u>. It is not intended for long-term use because it is <u>not effective for muscle spasms beyond 2–3 weeks.</u> It is not useful for spasticity due to neurologic conditions such as cerebral palsy.

Flexeril is not used for the treatment of depression, but it has the structure of a <u>tricyclic</u> antidepressant (TCA) by structure. It differs from amitriptyline (Elavil) by just one double bond. Flexeril causes similar side effects as TCAs, but is much <u>less dangerous</u> in overdose. Of 209 cyclobenzaprine overdose cases, there were no deaths and the QT interval was not prolonged (Bebarta et al, 2011).

Flexeril reduces spasticity through central action, possibly at the brainstem level. It is a 5-HT$_2$ antagonist that reduces muscle tone by decreasing activity of descending serotonergic neurons. Amitriptyline (Elavil) and cyproheptadine (Periactin) have been shown to do this also (Honda et al, 2003).

Dynamic interactions are similar to those of TCAs.

Cyclobenzaprine can theoretically contribute to <u>serotonin syndrome</u> when combined with other serotonergics and is contraindicated with monoamine oxidase inhibitors (MAOIs). However, the risk is very low.

> **Cyclobenzaprine is highly <u>unlikely</u> to contribute to serotonin syndrome.**

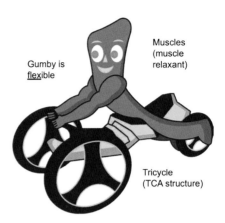

Gumby is <u>flex</u>ible

Muscles (muscle relaxant)

Tricycle (TCA structure)

Kinetic interactions with cyclobenzaprine differ from interactions with TCAs. Cyclobenzaprine is a 1A2 substrate (tree) while all TCA antidepressants are 2D6 substrates (beach balls).

Incidence of <u>drowsiness</u> with cyclobenzaprine is 38%. As with some TCAs, cyclobenzaprine can be used as a sleep medication due to its effects on 5-HT$_{2A}$, alpha-1 adrenergic, and H$_1$ histamine receptors. Flexeril causes anticholinergic side effects, but less so than carisoprodol (Soma) or tizanidine (Zanaflex). None of these spasmolytics should be taken by elderly individuals.

When taken orally, first-pass metabolism in the liver converts much of the dose to norcyclobenzaprine, which is more responsible for the persistent grogginess of the drug. Tonix Pharmaceuticals was testing sublingual cyclobenzaprine for military-related PTSD at 2.8 mg and 5.6 mg strengths, but the trial was halted in Phase III (2018) due to inadequate separation from placebo.

Although it only works short-term as a muscle relaxant, some patients take cyclobenzaprine long-term for insomnia.

Dosing: For muscle spasms the recommended dose is 5–<u>10 mg</u> TID for up to 3 weeks. When used off-label for fibromyalgia, start 10 mg HS, with a maximum of 40 mg total daily dose divided BID–TID.

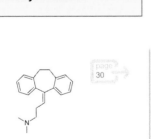

cyclobenzaprine (Flexeril)

amitriptyline (Elavil)

page 30 →

Dynamic interactions:
❖ Anticholinergic (moderate)
❖ Serotonergic (weak)
❖ Sedation/CNS depression
❖ Lowers seizure threshold

Kinetic interactions:
❖ 1A2 substrate

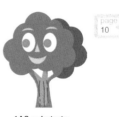

1A2 substrate

page 10 →

1953
$7–$11

Dextromethorphan (DXM)
dex troe meth OR fan

"Dexter the Thor fan"

❖ Cough suppressant
❖ Dissociative
❖ NMDA antagonist
❖ Sigma-1 agonist
❖ SRI

30 mg/
5 mL

FDA-approved for:

❖ Cough suppression

Used off-label for:

❖ Neuropathic pain
❖ Opioid withdrawal
❖ Postoperative pain
❖ Premature ejaculation
❖ Agitation of dementia

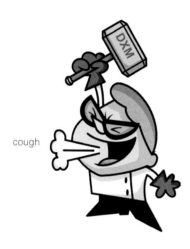

cough

Dextromethorphan (DXM) is an over-the-counter cough suppressant. It is kept behind the counter due to its dissociative properties, which lend to recreational use among young people. DXM is a component of Robitussin, NyQuil, Dimetapp, and Mucinex DM.

At high doses, DXM may produce euphoria and dissociative effects similar to ketamine. With prolonged use, psychological dependence is possible. It does not cause physical dependence, but can produce symptoms of antidepressant discontinuation syndrome owing to DXM's effects as a serotonin reuptake inhibitor (SRI).

In addition to being a SRI, DXM is an NMDA receptor antagonist and sigma-1 receptor agonist. Sigma-1 receptors in the limbic system of the brain may be involved in control of

emotions, possibly explaining the benefit of DXM for treatment of pseudobulbar affect (in combination with quinidine, which serves to extend half-life of DXM). An endogenous ligand for the sigma-1 receptor is yet to be identified, but we know some androgenic steroids activate the receptor.

Experimentally, DXM is being used to treat depression and negative symptoms of schizophrenia.

Dextromethorphan cough syrup is not to be confused with the cough syrup used to make "purple drank" (aka sizzurp), would is prescription-strength codeine and promethazine syrup. Unlike DXM, codeine can cause physical dependence.

DXM can contribute to serotonin syndrome.

Dynamic interactions:
❖ Serotonergic

Kinetic interactions:
❖ 2D6 substrate (major)

Dextromethorphan is a 2D6 substrate. When combined with a strong 2D6 inhibitor, its half-life is extended. This interaction is used for therapeutic effect by NUEDEXTA—a combination of DXM and quinidine (a strong 2D6 inhibitor).

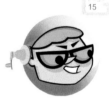

page 15

2D6 substrate

Serotonergic hallucinogens

Hallucinogens, also referred to as psychedelics, cause perceptual changes in a state of full wakefulness and alertness (as opposed to a state of delirium or sedation). It may be more accurate to refer to these drugs as "illusionogens" because their prominent effect is distortion or enhancement of existing stimuli (Abigail Herron, DO). The following hallucinogens can cause serotonin syndrome.

Hallucinogen	Mechanism	Comments
Lysergic acid diethylamide (LSD)	5-HT$_{2A}$ serotonin receptor agonist	Synthesized in 1938, not naturally occurring. Consumed by piece of blotter paper on the tongue; More info on subsequent page.
Dimethyltryptamine (DMT)	5-HT$_{2A}$ serotonin receptor agonist	Nicknamed "Dimitri" and "Businessman's Trip" due to short duration of about 1 hour; May be smoked; Tiny amounts are present endogenously, produced by the pineal gland.
Mescaline (peyote)	5-HT$_{2A}$ serotonin receptor agonist	Ingested as buttons from the crown of the peyote cactus; Lasts 4–8 hours; DEA Schedule I (illegal) with an exception for Native American religious ceremonies.
Psilocybin (mushrooms)	5-HT$_{2A}$ serotonin receptor agonist	"Magic mushrooms" or "shrooms"; Ingested for a trip lasting 4–6 hours; DEA Schedule I (illegal); May cause psychosis/detachment from reality; Reported mystical-like experiences
MDMA (Ecstasy, X, Molly)	Highly serotonergic, with stimulant and oxytocin-mediated effects	Described as a "psychedelic amphetamine" and "empathogen". Only 55% of users hallucinate; Extended duration; Altered perception of time (90%), euphoria (97%), increased awareness of emotions (50%), *decreased* impulsivity (25%), increased empathic connection to others due to oxytocin release from the pituitary. Can cause bruxism—it's the reason pacifiers are seen at raves; Risk of irreversible brain damage from massive release of serotonin. Risk of hyponatremia and toxidrome including rhabdomyolysis; The only hallucinogen with a defined withdrawal syndrome. "Molly" is powdered MDMA in a capsule; "Ecstasy" is a pressed pill. Both are commonly laced with other drugs.
Bufotenine	Serotonergic	Bufotenine has been consumed by licking toads of the genus *Bufo* or drinking their venom.

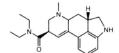 1943

Lysergic acid diethylamide (LSD)
"Lucy's Serotonergic Drug"

❖ Hallucinogen
❖ DEA Schedule I (illegal)
❖ 5-HT$_{2A}$ agonist

LSD can cause serotonin syndrome.

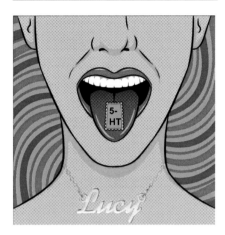

Although John Lennon denied that it is a drug song, the Beatles' '"Lucy in the Sky with Diamonds" is obviously about LSD.

Picture yourself in a boat on a river
With tangerine trees and marmalade skies
Somebody calls you, you answer quite slowly
A girl with kaleidoscope eyes…

Follow her down to a bridge by a fountain
Where rocking horse people eat marshmallow pies
Everyone smiles as you drift past the flowers
That grow so incredibly high

Lysergic acid diethylamide (LSD) is a semisynthetic product of lysergic acid, a natural substance from an ergot fungus. Referred to as "acid", LSD is a recreational hallucinogenic typically consumed in small doses on the tongue as blotter paper that was soaked in an LSD-containing solution and dried.

The hallucinogenic effect of LSD was discovered in 1943. It was a popular legal recreational drug in the early 1960s, but has been illegal since 1968.

LSD is gaining traction as a therapeutic drug. It has been found to treat and prevent cluster headaches and may work for treatment-resistant depression. Therapeutic effects may be achievable in micro doses that are sub-psychedelic (i.e., do not cause hallucinations). Even at psychedelic strength, LSD has minimal potential for addiction and may have potential as a treatment of addiction to other substances.

The effect of LSD is felt to be due entirely to prolonged stimulation of 5-HT$_{2A}$ serotonin receptors, which is the same mechanism of other classic hallucinogens like DMT, psilocybin and mescaline. These are the receptors blocked by many second generation antipsychotics (SGAs). Endogenous serotonin binds these receptors briefly, while LSD is essentially locked onto the receptor for hours. LSD is mostly cleared from the bloodstream within 6 hours, but the hallucinogenic effect continues for an average of 12 hours because this is how long LSD is stuck to a 5-HT$_{2A}$ receptor. Unsurprisingly, LSD can be a contributor to serotonin syndrome.

Overdose deaths on LSD alone are essentially non-existent, but are possible with 100–200x the usual dose. Terrifying "bad trips" are possible. Due to LSD's effects on the hypothalamus, it may elevate body temperature, raise blood pressure and make it virtually impossible to fall asleep while it is in effect.

Following cessation of LSD, the user may experience persisting perceptual disturbances as "LSD flashbacks", for instance seeing trails of moving objects, afterimages, or misperceptions of images as too large (macropsia) or too small (micropsia). Flashbacks may occur in individuals with minimal exposure to LSD. Flashbacks only constitute a disorder (Hallucinogen Persisting Perception Disorder, DSM-5) if they cause clinically significant distress or impairment.

LSD is regulated by the DEA as a Schedule I (illegal) controlled substance. Lysergic acid (without the 'D'), commonly known as ergine from morning glory seeds, has milder psychedelic properties and is Schedule III. Other lysergic acid derivatives include the dopaminergic agonist bromocriptine, and the headache medications ergotamine and methysergide.

For context, LSD's stimulation of 5-HT$_{2A}$ receptors is the opposite of what second-generation antipsychotics (SGAs) do. Mnemonic: 2A for 2nd Gen Antipsychotics, which block 5-HT$_{2A}$ receptors.

LSD has serotonin essentially embedded in its structure.

LSD   Serotonin

Dilated pupils are seen with LSD use and with serotonin syndrome, which can be caused by LSD .

Dynamic interactions:
❖ Serotonergic (strong)

Kinetic interactions:
❖ LSD is metabolized by 3A4 and other CYP enzymes.

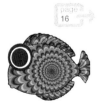

3A4 substrate

page 16

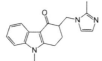

#91
1991
$3–$76 tab
$3–$76 ODT

Ondansetron (ZOFRAN)
on DAN se tron / ZO fran
"On Dancer Tron! (Go) so frantic!"

❖ Antiemetic
❖ Serotonin 5-HT$_3$ receptor antagonist

ODT	tab
4 8 mg	4 8 mg

FDA-approved for:
❖ Prevention of nausea/vomiting associated with:
  ❖ Chemotherapy
  ❖ Radiating therapy
  ❖ Surgery

Used off-label for:
❖ Nausea/vomiting (other)
❖ Irritable bowel syndrome
❖ Tourette's syndrome
❖ Schizophrenia (adjunct)
❖ Tardive dyskinesia
❖ Obsessive-compulsive disorder (OCD)
❖ Alcoholism

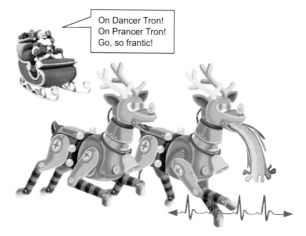

On Dancer Tron!
On Prancer Tron!
Go, so frantic!

QT prolongation
(intravenous route)

Ondansetron (Zofran) is the first-line medication for nausea/vomiting. It blocks the 5-HT$_3$ serotonin receptor, which is involved in antidepressant-induced nausea. Ondansetron's receptor binding profile is "clean", i.e., it does not bind off-target receptors like other antiemetics. Ondansetron exerts its effect in the gastrointestinal tract and in the brain's chemoreceptor trigger zone.

Ondansetron is a more effective antiemetic than dopamine blockers such as metoclopramide (Reglan). Another advantage over metoclopramide is ondansetron's lack of extrapyramidal effects (EPS) and sedation. It does not work well for nausea due to motion sickness, which is better treated with an anticholinergic like diphenhydramine, promethazine, or scopolamine.

Ondansetron is very well-tolerated. It can be somewhat constipating. Otherwise, no side effects are expected.

In 2011 the FDA issued a warning about ondansetron causing QT prolongation, although this is not a black box warning. QT prolongation is not much of an issue with oral ondansetron. In 2012 the 32 mg IV dose was withdrawn due to QT prolongation. The maximum IV dose is now 16 mg. The maximum PO dose is 24 mg.

Ondansetron is available as an orally disintegrating tablet (ODT), branded as ONDISSOLVE, which costs no more than the swallowed tablet. The ODT formulation can be taken sublingually for faster onset of action.

An effective regimen for preventing vomiting from cancer chemotherapy is a combination of a "-setron" and the corticosteroid dexamethasone (Decadron). How corticosteroids prevent vomiting is unclear.

Antidepressant-induced nausea

Nausea is one of the most common reasons patients stop medications prematurely. Nausea tends to be a transient side effect that usually resolves spontaneously. Nausea can often be avoided altogether with slow titration. Other tips for medication-induced nausea is to take the pill after food—not with food, but immediately after a meal. Also effective for nausea is ginger extract (one 550 mg capsule) taken 1 hour before a meal, for a maximum of 3 caps/day (Bodagh et al, 2019; Rajnish Mago, MD; The Carlat Psychiatry Report, Jun/Jul 2019). Ginger ale does not suffice.

Ondansetron may have value in the treatment of schizophrenia, as an adjunct to haloperidol (Zhang et al, 2006). Ondansetron has been proposed as a possible treatment for psychosis associated with Parkinson's disease (Zoldan et al, 1995). The mechanism of ondansetron's purported antipsychotic effect is unknown. It does not block dopamine receptors like traditional antipsychotics. It does not significantly block the 5-HT$_{2A}$ receptor that is targeted by second generation antipsychotics and pimavanserin (Nuplazid). If ondansetron is proven to truly benefit schizophrenia, the etiology of psychosis may need to be reconsidered.

Ondansetron could possibly improve tardive dyskinesia (Zullino et al, 2001).

Similar serotonin receptor antagonist ("-setron") antiemetics include granisetron (Kytril), palonosetron (Aloxi), and dolasetron (Anzemet). Other chemicals that have antiemetic properties due to blocking 5-HT$_3$ receptors are ginger and mirtazapine (Remeron). The antidepressant vortioxetine (Trintellix) blocks 5-HT$_3$ receptors but may cause nausea by other serotonergic mechanisms.

Dosing: The orally disintegrating tablet (ODT) formulation is preferred. The standard dose for nausea/vomiting is around **4 mg q 4 hr PRN** or **8** mg q **8** hr PRN. Scheduled dosing usually starts at 4 mg TID before meals. The maximum IV dose is 16 mg, limited due to QT prolongation. The maximum PO dose is 24 mg. For experimental psychiatric uses such as OCD and alcoholism, very low doses were used, for instance 0.25 mg BID for two weeks, then increased to 0.5 mg BID (Pallanti et al, 2013 for OCD).

Dynamic interactions:
❖ QT prolongation
❖ Anti-serotonergic - potential for profound hypotension in combination with apomorphine (Apokyn)

Kinetic interactions:
❖ 3A4 substrate

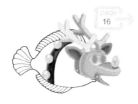

3A4 substrate

1961	
$14–$30	

Cyproheptadine (PERIACTIN)

si pro HEP tuh deen / pear e ACT in

"Perry actin'…help to dine"

❖ 1st Generation antihistamine
❖ Anticholinergic
❖ 5-HT₂ serotonin receptor antagonist

4 mg

FDA-approved for:
❖ Allergic rhinitis
❖ Urticaria

Used off-label for:
❖ Appetite stimulation
❖ Serotonin syndrome
❖ Female anorgasmia
❖ Nightmares
❖ Akathisia
❖ SSRI-induced sweating

Cyproheptadine (Periactin), released in 1961, is a first generation antihistamine with antiserotonergic properties. As with all first generation antihistamines, cyproheptadine is highly anticholinergic.

Cyproheptadine is FDA-approved as an antihistamine for allergic rhinitis and urticaria but is not used for these conditions because it causes a lot of weight gain. Cyproheptadine is useful as an appetite stimulant off-label.

Cyproheptadine's antiserotonergic effects can oppose the action of antidepressants, potentially rendering them ineffective. Nonetheless, it has been used to counteract SSRI-induced night sweats. Cyproheptadine can be used as a treatment for serotonin syndrome, though the main intervention is stopping the serotonergic culprit(s).

Cyproheptadine is used off-label to treat nightmares. Unless the patient needs to gain weight, prazosin (Minipress) and gabapentin (Neurontin) should be tried before resorting to cyproheptadine.

Cyproheptadine is also used off-label for treatment of female anorgasmia. Serotonergics (e.g., SSRIs) may cause anorgansmia, so it makes sense that an antiserotonergic could facilitate orgasm.

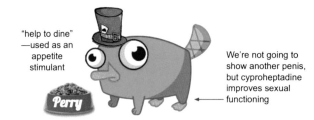

"help to dine" —used as an appetite stimulant

We're not going to show another penis, but cyproheptadine improves sexual functioning

Perry Actin'—In the cartoon Phineas and Ferb, Perry the Platypus is a crime-fighting spy, but is often undercover actin' like a docile pet. For Perry to act like a pet, it would help to dine on pet food.

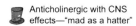 Anticholinergic with CNS effects—"mad as a hatter"

Dosing: To stimulate appetite start 2 mg QID and increase to target dose of 8 mg QID over 3 weeks. For serotonin syndrome give 12 mg x 1, then 2 mg q 2 hr until response (max 32 mg/day). To treat female anorgasmia, the dose is 4–12 mg PRN 1–2 hr prior to sex. For nightmares, start 4 mg HS but may need to go as high as 24 mg HS; Although cyproheptadine is no longer used for the FDA-approved indications of allergic rhinitis and urticaria, the dose would be 4 mg TID.

The structure of cyproheptadine is closely related to tricyclic antidepressants (TCAs), but cyproheptadine is antiserotonergic, not serotonergic like a TCA.

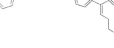

cyproheptadine (Periactin)   amitriptyline (Elavil) - TCA

Dynamic interactions:
❖ Antiserotonergic effects can oppose therapeutic effects of serotonergic antidepressants.
❖ Sedative
❖ Anticholinergic
  – constipation
  – confusion
  – urinary retention
  – dry mouth

Kinetic interactions:
❖ None significant

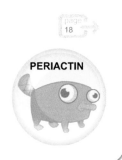

PERIACTIN

page 18 →

About the author:

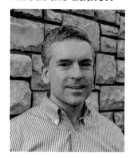

Dr Jason Cafer is Medical Director for Behavioral Health Services at SSM Health/St. Mary's Hospital in Jefferson City, Missouri where he serves as attending physician for a bustling 20-bed acute inpatient psychiatric ward. He graduated from University of Missouri-Columbia School of Medicine in 2003 and completed Psychiatric Residency at the same institution in 2007. He is a diplomate of the American Board of Psychiatry and Neurology and is also board-certified in Addiction Medicine by the American Board of Preventive Medicine. Prior to St. Mary's, he practiced inpatient psychiatry at Fulton State Hospital and outpatient at Comprehensive Health Systems. In 2007 he founded Iconic Health, a medical informatics startup that obtained angel round funding. He was Principal Investigator for Phase I and II Small Business Innovation Research (SBIR) grants for "Online Rural Telepsychiatry Platform" (2007-2009) funded by the United States Department of Agriculture. He is the inventor of United States Patent US8255241B2 which was the subject of an SBIR grant awarded by the Department of Health and Human Services for "Medication IconoGraphs: Visualization of Complex Medication Regimens". He completed *Cafer's Psychopharmacology* while serving as preceptor for Stephens College Master of Physician Assistant Studies program.

Visualize to Memorize
Psychopharmacology

also available:

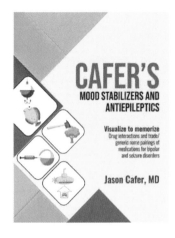

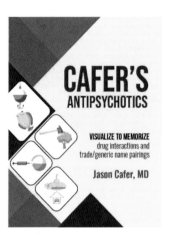

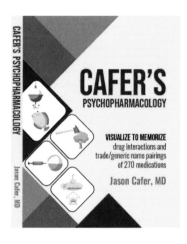

Cafer's Mood Stabilizers and Antiepileptics
39 medications

Cafer's Antipsychotics
40 medications

Cafer's Psychopharmacology
270 medications

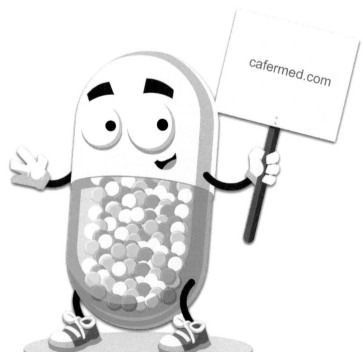

Cafermed.com discount code for
*Cafer's Psychopharmacology:
Visualize to Memorize 270
Medication Mascots:* **EMBIGGEN**

Made in the USA
Coppell, TX
09 May 2021